PHYSICAL RESULTS
The Most Direct Route!

PHYSICAL RESULTS
The Most Direct Route!

By

Brad L. Nachtigal

ISBN 1-58500-890-7

1st Books-rev. 9/22/00

INTRODUCTION

GET THE LOOK!

GET *PHYSICAL* RESULTS

STRIP THE FAT, BUILD INCREDIBLY LEAN MUSCLE
30-50% FASTER than anything you have tried before,
by learning the secrets of *The Most Direct Route.*
SEE results in 30 - 60 days
FEEL it *Immediately*

It is doubtful you have ever experienced anything like it!

Americans are no longer in the dark where health and fitness are concerned. They are fed up with hype and promises that have become either gimmick-ridden or completely unrealistic. The student/athlete, teacher, weekend warrior, or housewife, all want nothing more than to simply know **WHAT WORKS** and **HOW TO GET THERE.** That's it!

Unfortunately, the message still being sent remains frustratingly unclear, **YOU'RE STILL NOT GETTING IT!** Not the eating part of it, not the exercise part, and as a whole, hardly any part of getting fit. WHY?

Why do those truly devoted to making a positive change in their lives always find themselves asking just this question? ***WHY?***

I have found that so many times when it comes to health and fitness, one eventually finds that effort alone will not always yield and produce results. Instead, one needs a specific map to follow. A map that will accurately guide one around all possible detours and wrong turns. A confident, reassuring notion of travelling the right road towards physical success.

Introducing, PHYSICAL RESULTS. A straight and to the point problem-solver aimed directly at getting results, plain and simple. Nothing too fancy, too complicated or over-bearing.

Just what you need to know, to get you where you want, that's it!

If you're not **getting** it now, you will! If you're not **feeling** it now, you will! If you're not **thinking** it now, you will! Once you start and get into it, there can be no stopping you.

Physical Results will emphasize, primarily, in the direction of body SCULPTING by way of the most direct route. Not always the simplest OR the hardest, but *THE most direct route.* Looking and getting that well proportioned, defined, ripped look, with the burning off of unsightly fat.

Because now, more than ever, *LEAN* is where it's at. Most people don't have the need or desire to become a Mr. or Mrs. Universe, sporting huge bulging muscles, thus requiring grueling hours of daily workouts combined with extreme dieting, drugs and so on. For most of us, this combination of fitness overkill along with the average day-to-day lifestyle becomes very impractical. We need something tolerably in between.

Physical Results will give you that choice, given a little honest work, dedication and sacrifice.

It is, also, not something I would ask of someone and not do myself. I practice what I preach. (Just try asking that of some of our doctors, physicians, or so-called health experts about that one!)

As a former 3-time All-American, 2-time Olympic hopeful, personal fitness trainer, and at present, full-time farmer, fire fighter and parent, I feel as though I've seen it all. I've spent the last twenty years listening to people of all ages, from all walks of life, talk about their concerns and complaints, their questions and their conclusions. But mainly, I have found it to be their genuine feelings of *frustration* that cries out the loudest.

Like most of you, I too, know the problems and setbacks associated with coming up short of my goals at a time when I want them the most. Those primary stumbling blocks that keep even the most determined individuals' fitness goals just out of fingertip reach. Yet, a distance that can finally be bridged .... via the answers that lie here in this book.

Granted, there are certain similarities between this and other success-proven programs, ***HOWEVER, this one is unmatched in other ways that make this particular approach stand very much alone.*** Check this out!

First, each of the *most direct route* concepts are explained in layman's terms most anyone can understand, **leaving out the body chemistry and technical jargon 99 per cent of you probably wouldn't care about anyway.** Everything is straight and to the point.

Secondly, this is **NOT** a weight loss program. It IS a **Fat Loss** program. Here, the differences will be measured by what exactly is taken off and how long the effects actually last.

Thirdly, only ***the* most beneficial exercises** have been chosen for you. Each particular exercise is specifically chosen because of its proven effectiveness in providing *accelerated results.*

This **abbreviated** approach dramatically eliminates the confusion factor, unlike other programs that continue to keep stacking them on. Here, you will not find 101 ways to do a sit-up or 10 ways to a better bicep. Such additional time-consuming methods **are no longer necessary.**

Fourth, each exercise is purposefully placed in a specific order that maximizes your precious time and effort. This type of program helps by **cutting the usual number of exercises** it would normally take to do the same job.

Fifth, a quite unique, and one-of-it's-kind, "Troubleshooting" section is provided towards the end of the book for your convenience. **In book form, this is as close to a personal trainer as one can get.** At one's fingertips is a step-by-step problem solving guide that will not only deliver the physical goods, but just as importantly, strengthen your mental problem solving abilities in the process.

"Troubleshooting" is based upon specialized tricks-of-the-trade, compiled from many years of exercise experience and a lot of trial and error. *There is nothing like it anywhere!*

Sixth, this particular approach to fitness directly trains your *mind* as well as your body, enabling you to be **totally and independently complete.** Because if you don't truly understand what is taking place on the inside, trust me, you will find little accomplished on the outside.

Seventh, what makes everything finally come together and click will be learning the concepts of **"M.E.T."**, which stands for *Maximum Efficiency Training.*

This will eliminate any and all wasted time and effort of this particular weight training program, *in comparison to all others*. Here, I reveal secret techniques few know about and even fewer have mastered, not so much by what is said, but HOW it is presented.

You will also find many other *most direct route* approaches, ones that *simply* and *systematically* teach you such things as **long-term weight control** (eating simply by simply eating), through learning how to become independently self-sufficient, both in and outside our world of fitness.

"Physical Results" *is a COMPLETE mind/body system* **that will continue to work year after year, long after the trend-setting quick fixes have come and gone.**

Whatever the problem, whatever the desire, goals large or small, for the young or old, by following and implementing this **self-solving** approach to fitness and well-being, the odds are highly in your favor that you too, will finally expose your own personal "missing link" to physical success. A link that comes to many as **a real eye-opener.**

When it happens, you'll know it. And when you do, you'll then learn to recognize it, decipher it, and then conquer it.

Take---this---book---seriously, and then watch what happens!

TABLE OF CONTENTS

ACKNOWLEDGEMENTS

I would like first and foremost thank the good Lord for blessing me with the best parents a guy could ever have. Thanks Ann and Roy for your overwhelming love and support in everything I have done over my first 40 years of life. If not for you, this book probably would not have been possible. To you both, I will never be able to thank enough.

To my three brothers, Kelly, Steve, and David, all have provided additional support, encouragement, and a lot of patience in putting up with me and my sometimes idealistic ways.

I cannot express strongly enough, my feelings of gratitude and how very lucky I have been to be blessed with such a wonderful family. One could not have been luckier. I humbly thank you all!

Also, to my good friend and former coach David Johnston, who unselfishly took me under his wing, provided support, and kicked me in the behind just when I needed it most. You were always there for me, always an inspiration, and will always be my friend. Thanks bud!

A special thanks to Richard Seck. A fellow farmer, neighbor, and close friend. One who would drop whatever he happened to be doing at the time to help a friend in need. I can always count on you for advice and guidance, whether it be in farming or computers. If it hadn't been for you, I would still be trying to bang out something resembling a manuscript on some old typewriter.

I would also like to thank my brother David Nachtigal, sister-in-law Kim Nachtigal, Alison Brown-Ubert, the "Hutchinson Racquet And Fitness Club", and of course, Don Siedhoff of "Rock Island Studio Photography", for their parts in the illustration of this book.

Last and most importantly I would like to thank my wife Angie, for her never-ending support and blessing me with two of the greatest gifts a man could ever have, Haylee and Cade.

PREFACE

Before you go any further I feel the need to forewarn you. In reading this book you may, at times, feel as though I come down a little hard on certain groups of people and/or types of individuals. Please believe me when I say it is never my intention to hurt feelings or convey pessimism. This book is not about singling anyone out by any means.

But by the same token, it is not in my nature to pull punches or blow smoke. I simply tell it like it is. For it has been my experience that for many, some kind of trigger mechanism somewhere deep within each of us has to be pulled in order to get one to act. I say again, to **get you to act**. There may be other ways to go about getting results but what I apparently lack in finesse, you will come to find I more than make up for it in substance.

I can promise you that if you stay with me and remain true to your quest, **YOU WILL** reap that which you seek!

Also, though I have done my best to provide you with what I refer to as *the most direct route* towards acquiring a lean, fit mind and body, you will at times come across concepts that seem somewhat redundant and at best, more like *the longest route possible*. But understand this, everything mentioned must be approached openly and patiently. **Long term success**, which is what I promote, must have some kind of fitness-oriented <u>foundation</u> from which to draw from when you finally begin to initiate the actual programs and techniques provided here in this book.

Once you achieve the proper mindset and knowledge base required, the path toward your goals will become clear and complete.

*************DISCLAIMER*************

And finally, although I continually stress the safety aspect throughout this book, there will always be those who feel bulletproof and venture far outside that of their own physical limitations.

Therefore, I must state that neither the author, publisher, or anyone related to the production of this book be held liable for any and all mishaps that may happen.

****

STEP I:

WISE UP!

CHAPTER ONE:

EXERCISE EDUCATION, A FAILING GRADE?

YOU STILL AREN'T GETTING IT ARE YOU? There are just way too many of you that strive to become physically fit but either;

- Don't know how,
- Do know how, but don't try or,
- Do it anywhere from slightly to all wrong.

What's the catch? What's the mystery? Why can some do it while so many others can't? Just what's the big secret?

Is it because the source pool is all dried up? Nothing of value out there that teaches us all the how-to's? No one to ask or confide in? Has our health community completely let us down?

The answer.....not in the least! Actually, there has been more overkill on the topic of health and fitness by way of books, magazines, TV info-mercials, videos, sports, celebrity endorsements, and the glorifying nature of other media propaganda. Simply put, we, as average run-of-the-mill individuals, have run into the insurmountable task of having to sift through it all, in an often vain attempt to find what really works. And I mean, *what really works!* Not just for Joe or Jane working-class, but what works for the student, non-professional athlete, the non-professional bodybuilder and so on.

The fact is, those of us that do fall into this category of mainstream are usually not much of an expert in such fields of fitness. That is why the majority of us look elsewhere for answers. Answers, that many times, come in the form of short-term fixes, gimmicks, and even program overkill on numerous diet and exercise schemes.

So, who is to blame? You, or the health-crazed educational system in which we live? If there was a grading system that could be given for this particular class we shall call: "Fitness 101", the report card would probably look something like this:

- I give our health field experts an A minus for their efforts in trying to educate us as a whole. They do a fairly good job, sometimes too good a job, an overload of numerous facts, figures and studies. A noble effort, but at times, quite overwhelming while losing many of us in the process.

- I give our pill-popping, gimmick-inventing, exercise entrepreneurs a D for preying on the weak and trusting in an attempt to reach their only goal, that of getting rich.

- But, I give most of those out there who DO want to change and better themselves health-wise, a big fat F. That's right, a failing grade. If the desire is truly there, whatever one may require IS out there. One need only to have the gumption to go out and find the right answers, then follow through. A trait that bears no fault to anyone but themselves.

To put it bluntly, it is ultimately up to YOU to look after your own health and well-being regardless of the circumstances. From this point forward, instead of constantly leaning on someone, something, or some program, it's you that must take the responsibility for getting your own (exercise) education. No excuses! In other words, *lean more towards learning, rather than being so quick as in learning to lean!*

Only until you honestly look at yourself in the mirror and face the real reasons you are where you are, then and only then, will you be ready to move forward. If you can't even do this, then you're only fooling yourself.

Even if you're capable of coming to terms with that reflection in the mirror, there are other pre-requisites that must first be addressed before you are eligible to receive any passing grade. Early fitness pre-requisites that will ultimately decide whether or not you pass or fail.

a) Wise up! Don't be like so many who continue to take the stand, **If there is an easier route to take, take it first**. The majority of those who fail in health and fitness are those who kid themselves into truly believing that next to nothing is all that is required. WRONG!

b) Wise up! Just because something touted **new** or **state-of-the-art** comes along, does not mean everything up to that point immediately gets thrown out the window. Much of the successful, time-proven, basic fundamentals too often take a back seat in favor of the deceptive quick and easy fix. However, it usually doesn't take long to find that this fad or ride on the bandwagon is bumpy and short-lived. It is an uncertain path that begins with hope, yet all too often ends in failure.

c) Wise up! Finally getting that body you want is never just a *physical* accomplishment. Those who succeed have done so only because they have grown mentally as well. Self-confidence, self-esteem, and self-sufficiency, all happen to be subliminal by-products of exercise that are usually not considered during the early goal setting stages.

d) Wise up! Exercise should be made to be as enjoyable as possible under the circumstances, at least that's what many experts will tell you. But in real life, exercise should be accepted for what it really is, *DEMANDING!* An exerted effort on you're part. Remember, there is no effortless or comfortable way to get you where you want, **in anything**. Accepting this from the very beginning moves you one step closer to success.

With the <u>understanding</u> *and* <u>acceptance</u> of these pre-req.'s out of the way, it's now time for the actual course to begin. But, before any problems can be solved, *you must first have the answers.*

Therefore, as was just mentioned in the preface, it is my deliberate intention to re-submit certain criteria throughout early portions of this book that I feel not enough of you are getting, *understanding*, or *accepting*, regardless of the source. And yes, some of which you will recognize, while some you may not.   In either case, everything mentioned is vital to *the most direct route* concept and should not be skipped over.

Simply start from the beginning and work your way through each chapter in the order given, even though specific goals and interests may lie elsewhere. As you will soon learn, long lasting success in health and fitness is never a one-track, one-sided approach, rather, it becomes more of a multi-dimensional combination of several components, working as one.

Now, pay attention, sit up straight, and open your book to Chapter two, "What's Up Doc?" For if your efforts are really true and sincere towards achieving a certain degree of health, fitness, and well-being, then this is your opportunity to finally make that passing grade in this seemingly never-ending plight called, "Exercise Education." This time, let's *really* do it!

CHAPTER TWO:

WHAT'S UP DOC?

Health and Fitness, a seemingly endless quest for those who want it all, yet few ever find. A void that embodies over 85% of the American society today.

What makes this scenario even worse, is that we are all reminded of it every day. Family, friends, doctors, magazines, and television, are among the generous portion of authority figures that are either directly or indirectly involved with influencing the way we standardize and measure our health.

Typically, what is good health and how do you know when you've reached it? It's not hard to recognize or feel what it's like to be out of shape, but at what point will you finally realize that you have reached a sufficient level of fitness to be classified as good or even excellent shape? Is it when you are able to run a four minute mile? Is it measured on how much weight you are able to bench press? How many pounds you were able to shed? Or, finally, collecting those Ohh's and Ahh's from all those around you? Just when or how does one know?

It is with these questions in mind and at this early point in the book that I make this suggestion, **consult your doctor or physician BEFORE and DURING this or any other health and fitness program.**

No one individual is the same, each person has different goals, body makeup, and intensity levels. This creates a wide variation of possible injuries, among a multitude of other health related problems that should first be considered before undergoing any type of physical exertion. Some you should be aware of are as follows;

- High or low blood pressure
- History of, or susceptibility to heart attack
- Severe obesity
- Arthritis
- Dizzy spells
- Lower back and spinal problems
- Little or no flexibility
- Malnutrition
- Breathing problems
- Severe headaches
- Pain or swelling of the joints
- Diabetes and other such metabolic disorders

I'll bet your saying WHOA, wait just a minute. I've got one or all of these, and some not even on the list!

Well don't panic yet. Many of the concepts in this book can be done in spite of certain health problems, BUT only when used with extreme care, common sense, and with the professional advice of your personal physician.

Generally, most physicians encourage exercise to their patients who want to better their health. Hence, it will be these same medically trained individuals that will prove most beneficial in helping you determine which of the preceding exercises that will best fit your individual needs and capabilities. Exercises that will provide many life long benefits to those who put forth the effort. Listed here are many such examples of the ever-growing list.

BENEFITS OF EXERCISE

- increased capacity for work
- increased endurance
- increased lung capacity
- increased resistance against diseases
- increased joint flexibility
- increased bone mass and strength
- increased vigor
- increased ability to cope and handle stress
- increased physical strength
- increased body metabolism
- improved cardiovascular fitness
- improved digestion and bowel function
- improved physical coordination and neuromuscular skills
- improved sleep, rest, and relaxation
- improved attitude, mood, and feeling of well-being
- improved sexual function
- improved ability to cope with environmental hazards that come with such life activities as walking or driving
- improved mind-body relationship, which brings with it more self confidence, a better self image, and a positive approach to life as a whole
- improved recreational and athletic abilities
- lowered blood pressure
- lowered resting heart rate
- reduction of blood cholesterol and triglycerides
- faster reaction times
- slows the process of deterioration, aging

- decreases various anxiety conditions such as headache, backache, and insomnia, and depression
- decreases fatigue level
- better overall health rating

WHY ASK WHY?

While you are at the doctors' office be sure to ask any and all questions you may have about your role in the health and fitness world, and just what is in your best interest. In other words, be prepared to ask questions, writing them down if you have to. You've paid good money for the visit, so get all you can out of it. The doctor and his or her staff is there for you, not the other way around.

Such queries could include information about a possible eating schedule that best fits you. Let the doctor in on the physical goals and intensity levels you have set for yourself, and how it will relate to the nutritional requirements that must be met.

In addition to seeking advice about specific exercises and diet, other considerations you need to know are;

- your resting heart rate
- your hearts' respective training zone
- your maximum exercise heart rate (more important as age increases)

This is especially important to those who undertake more of an aerobic workout, such as jogging, biking, swimming, and so on. Most anyone can acquire this and other pertinent information through related charts, graphs, or various books and articles. But again, it is your doctor who can better provide you with a more personal guide to physical health regarding you, as an individual. (This is all covered later on in the chapter called "Aerobically Speaking".)

REFERRALS

If you presently don't have, or know of a good doctor, try the referral method, commonly known as word-of-mouth. Ask a friend or someone whose judgement you trust to give you a name or two. Such personal experiences can be a fairly reliable method of choosing just the right person, the one to whom you are about to entrust your body to.

Or, you may now choose from any one of a growing number of computerized services on the Internet that conveniently provide sound, reputable, medical referrals quickly and easily. Just such a personal referral or specialized service, is how many hospitals and private practices stay productive and prosperous. Without them, it would be hard to distinguish between the good one's, the so-so's, or the one's you would likely hesitate to take your pet hamster to.

Even if a particular physician cannot help directly, you will find most informally belong to sort of an elite, close-knit fraternity pool, in turn, having access to a wide array of referrals right at their fingertips. In other words, if they can't help, they can probably find someone who can.

All in all, always check first with your doctor before attempting anything new or different regarding diet or exercise. You know your doctor, and he knows you. He knows all about your body, both it's needs and it's vices. Yours is a relationship not just restricted to the office visit, but that of a valued friend. One with whom you can call on short notice, to listen, console, or advise you. The knowledge they possess is available to any and all, a virtual self-contained library of helpful information that could make many decisions on your health matters much easier to understand and live with. All you have to do is just ask!

CHAPTER THREE:

JUST SAY NO!

Unfortunately, there is still a vast majority out there who still subject their bodies to various mechanisms of destruction. Again, the indulgence of short-term highs like Steroids, Smoking, Alcohol, and Drugs, continue to take their toll in our society today. That's right, CONTINUE!

Even after years of study and research, fact upon fact, adults and children alike, knowingly use and abuse what is probably the most precious gift one could ever, ever have, ...their health.

Although total numbers and percentages have somewhat declined, there is still a large contingency of those who continue to indulge. Sadly, most are aware of the dire consequences that occur when partaking in such activities and habits, but choose, rather, to disregard the facts.

And so, for those who have somehow either missed the boat, need a refresher course, or simply were misinformed in one way or another, this chapter is for you. It is a blunt and deliberate wake up call for anyone on track to better health and well being. For those involved, it all begins here!

STEROIDS

(I apologize for the length and duration of this next subject-matter. It is my intention at this time, rather to educate than to instruct due to the important nature of the topic.)

For those already familiar with steroid use and its effects, this next section may or may not be for you. Regardless of the circumstances, you have already made your choice and are presently having to live with it now.

The following topic is primarily directed to those kids or young adults that are considering the use of steroids, due to peer pressure, athletics, curiosity, desperation or whatever the reason may be. I feel there <u>has</u> to be some way to get through to the prospective steroid user before it becomes too late and irreparable damage is done.

Quite simply, anabolic steroids are primarily male hormones that are used by an individual, to benefit or aid in the muscle building process. They have been known to increase one's muscle size, strength, and recuperative abilities at a faster rate than what would be considered normal, much like a magic potion or pill.

Although numerous studies have already been done and with the end seemingly no where in sight, the results of the long term effects are still not 100% fully known. You have probably come across such articles stemming from all kinds of various publications ranging from reputable medical journals, all the way down to your local newspaper. They all show possible side-effects from steroids as frightening and *real*. Whether you accept it or not, **they are** present at all levels, from the professional/amateur scene, on down through our high schools, and now even in our grade schools. Yes, in our grade schools!

A prime example of "proof after the fact", could be the way cigarettes and other tobacco products have been misused for so long. For many years it was socially acceptable to smoke without regard to any health risks. It was the "in" thing to do. Although there were studies being done at the time, there was *no official* recognition of smoking posing a hazard to health.

Unfortunately, thousands of people died (and are still dying) before it was finally confirmed. Many more developed lung cancer and unbreakable habits as a result. So what do we do now? Are we going to let yesterday repeat itself? Just when will we draw the line. Or perhaps better put, how deep shall the line be drawn? So far, society has shown it to be easier to turn and look the other way, only willing to admit partial acknowledgment of how bad it really is.

How long should we continue to allow our high school and college athletes to dose their bodies with steroids and other growth-enhancing chemicals before the experts tell us they finally have absolute proof of the harmful effects? How long should we wait for confirmation? How long should we wait before more bodies are ruined?

Have I ever used them? NO, not even tempted! I, personally, have NEVER in my life used or condoned the use of steroids, for the purpose of either gaining that competitive edge, or simply to look better in a mirror. Please, give me a break. What is this world coming to?

I am one of many that still believes that only through hard work and sacrifice is it possible to achieve that level of excellence that would propel one above the crowd. Not by the concept of cheating at all costs.

Using steroids just happens to be another form of <u>drug</u> use, period. It is for those who are weak and insecure in their own faith and abilities.

Those that argue this point often justify themselves by claiming steroids to be just another *training tool*, much the same way people use the new high-tech, state-of-the-art exercise machines, computer imaging, videos, and so on.

Wise up people, you don't get serious health problems like prostate cancer or shrinking of the testicles by using some fancy exercise machine or newly designed running shoe.

The essence and whole concept of weight training is for the betterment of health. So when one pumps drugs and steroids into their system, it unconditionally changes the entire meaning of health and fitness, ending up totally opposite of what sport is all about.

THE ETHICAL QUESTION

This quote taken from an article by T. Murray, "Get On With Sports, Leave Steroids Behind", best expresses those feelings and beliefs carried not only by myself, but that of an ever growing, determined cast of health-bound Americans.

"The ethical point of view of such drug use in sport has been described this way:

If I said I could put the shot 90 feet with the aid of a sling or 2 miles with a cannon, you would rightly tell me I have missed the point of sport?

If your opponent entered a swim meet with a jet ski, or a bicycle race with a motorcycle, you would contest this as giving him an unfair advantage? Drugs are the same kind of artificial manipulation of sport performance.

To put it another way;

In our conception of excellence in sport, some things are permissible, like expert coaching or exercise machines, and some things are not, like springs in shoes or drug-aided performance."

The odds were heavily against me as a Kansas farm boy who moved to the big city in the quest of making the Olympic team. I had no financial backing, little coaching, and was constantly challenged just to find adequate practice facilities and equipment. I didn't need the added burden of competing against those who chose the steroid route and other performance-enhancing drugs.

COMPETITION RUN AMOK

But can the competition really be that fierce? Do big contracts and big dollar signs play that important a role in the decision making process? Do many of our athletes, students, boys and girls next door really think it's worth the risk? Sadly, the answer is "Yes" on numerous accounts.

Some don't care what the risks are, even though the gains are relatively short-lived. But many others feel in order to stay competitive, they must join those who use them, regardless of their own personal fears and beliefs. The pressure one can be under to consistently perform at a top level is at times, just too much. It is widely agreed, that there needs to be a more suitable and accurate policing system, and soon!

In bodybuilding and track and field meets for example, there is now drug testing at many of the major competitions. Testing has also become mandatory in most college athletic programs, and even now with a growing number of high schools. Successful or not, it is at least an effort by some to try and clean up the reputation of sports and athletics if not for health reasons, but for the spirit of fair play.

YOU'RE OUTTA HERE

If an athlete chooses the path of steroids as a tool for that competitive edge, fine then, that's his or her choice. This is a free country. That particular individual will then be responsible for their own health risks. They alone will be the ones to suffer, during, and long after their competitive days are over.

HOWEVER, he or she will not be able to compete in any school athletics, or any other sports sanctioned programs. The use of anabolic steroids and like substances are on the list of banned doping substances of the USOC (United States Olympic Committee), IOC (International Olympic Committee), and NCAA (National Collegiate of Amateur Athletics) sports governing organizations. They have been declared ILLEGAL in our sports world, adding to ones like cocaine, marijuana, crack, and speed.

Let those individuals find their own competitions. Allow them to wear their own label of chemical freaks or fitness follies. Only then will it be clear cut in recognizing true physical talent and athletic achievement, through hard work, sacrifice, and dedication. The way it should always be.

RISK VS. SIDE-EFFECTS

This brings us down to the nitty gritty. If you thought your only worry using steroids was your conscience telling you "bad things only happen to the other guy", or "so what if I'm cheating a little", you could probably handle that, right? WRONG! The chances are **high** that you will experience at least one, and very possibly more of the side-effects listed. Examine and think carefully about each one, then ask yourself, is it worth the risk?

POSSIBLE SIDE-EFFECTS OF USING ANABOLIC STEROIDS

- CANCER
- HEART DISEASE
- LIVER MALFUNCTION
- LIVER TUMORS
- TESTICULAR ATROPHY, (shrinking of the testicles)
- REDUCED SPERM COUNT
- STERILITY
- MOOD CHANGES, some could be drastic
- GYNECOMASTIA, (the formation of female breast tissue in the male) Even if one decides to stop using, the condition could be such that surgery may be required to repair normality.
- BEHAVIORAL DISORDERS

- INCREASED AGGRESSIVENESS AND/OR HOSTILITY
- PREMATURE BALDNESS IN MEN AND WOMEN
- SEVERE ACNE ON FACE, BACK, AND SHOULDERS
- EXCESSIVE WATER RETENTION (BLOATED)
- PREMATURE STOPPING OF NORMAL BONE GROWTH in pre-adolescents- HIGH BLOOD PRESSURE- HYPERTENSION
- *** DEATH ***

THE SIDE EFFECTS ON THE FEMALE ARE EVEN MORE SEVERE

- MASCULINIZATION PROCESS INCREASED, could be permanent.
- FACIAL HAIR, at times quite noticeable and sometimes heavy
- MALE PATTERN BALDNESS
- MENSTRUAL CYCLE IRREGULARITY
- PERMANENT DEEPENING OF THE VOICE
- INCREASED SIZE OF FEMALE GENITALS
- UNKNOWN LONG TERM EFFECTS regarding child-bearing potential, fertility, reproductive organ cancer, and possible birth defects in offspring.
- ESPECIALLY DANGEROUS to those younger females who are either pre-pubertal or are not yet fully grown.

Still not convinced? Still feel lucky? Perhaps this would be a good time to take a moment to reflect back on the career of the late football great, All-Pro Defensive End, Lyle Alzado. Up until the end, he thought so too!

PSYCHOLOGICALLY SPEAKING – A VICIOUS CYCLE

Aside from the many health hazards listed, the possible physical, addictive processes, that seem to coincide with steroid use can be as much a vicious *cycle* to the _mind_, as it is to the *body*. And when you consider both afflictions together, compounding the ill-effects of both, steroid use creates a situation that is not only hard to break but hard to maintain any normal standard of health.

Again, we are talking about YOUR body. Not your friend, not some football player, not some guy or gal in a muscle magazine, YOURS.

The up-swing of steroid use has frequently been described as a "superman" type feeling. A sort of high that provides one with a greater sense of confidence, inner security, and even to a point of mental invincibility.

But, unfortunately, these feelings have been reached mainly by artificial means. Just as the typical drug user soon finds, what goes up, must eventually come back down. You cannot artificially stay up forever without falling deeper into the addiction.

This could then bring one to face to face with the other side of the coin, the down-swing.

During this downward spiral, one may go through various erratic and emotional mood swings, seemingly to have personality changes without reason. The user could also show signs of increased and uncontrolled aggressiveness, irritability, short-fused, or just an all-around more hostile and violent nature. Soon it becomes harder for those close to them to recognize the person they once knew. Relationships fail, family and friends tend to shy away.

If you or someone you know is contemplating using steroids, I recommend you read everything you can get your hands on regarding this topic, even dated material like "Death In The Locker Room", by Dr. Bob Goldman. It gives you something more to think about than the advice of your locker room buddies.

Sadly, if you think about it, it is very much a shame that there even exists a need for such a book, one regarding drug abuse prevention *for athletes*.

In closing this section on steroids, I found a frightfully amusing little story I would like to share with you. It was about a young man who approached a doctor in sports medicine, an authority on the topic of steroids. The young man asked the doctor if it would be OK to use anabolic steroids to aid him in achieving his goals. The doctor replied by telling him to reach down into his jeans, then ask himself if he really wants to tamper with what he's got down there.

ALCOHOL

Contrary to what you may have been told or how you feel about it, the consumption of alcohol has little or no benefit in regard to exercise and fitness. No thanks to all of those beer ads on television and in magazines, depicting sexy, young, vibrant bodies playing on the beach or pool side with a cool one in hand.

It's no wonder there is such a misconstrued, alcoholic attitude in this country today in an attempt, by some, to either directly or indirectly correlate fitness and fun with drinking.

Actually, various fitness level tests using alcohol consumption as the base, seem to show a decrease in dynamic muscular strength, balance, hand-eye coordination, and accuracy. How the so-called fun part enters into the equation is purely self-perceptual.

Nutritionally speaking, alcohol is more of a fat than that of a carbohydrate. The calories you get from drinking alcohol do not contribute positively towards better health, but rather contain many unwanted calories your body doesn't really need.

Having a beer or a drink on a regular basis is a major weakness for many who are trying to get back in shape. But, in order to achieve optimum physical goals quickly and efficiently, each must sacrifice such things and move diet and exercise far and above alcohol on their priority list.

So from now on, try and treat alcohol as you would any of the other so-called vices in life. You know, those everyday, life-entertaining, unhealthful habits like smoking, inactivity, and eating high fat foods.

SMOKING

If you have half a brain you should know by now that there is no place for smoking anywhere, at any time, especially where fitness is concerned. Simply put, smoking is OUT. It is no longer the "in" thing to do.

With the combined help of the Surgeon General and a steam-rolling, health-oriented society, smokers have now found themselves confined to a class all their own. Designated smoking areas, non-smoking flights, and banned smoking privileges in most indoor public and private places have all since taken place. Smokers rights have diminished to the extent that more and more are being shunned and singled out, in turn, restricting the actions of a few, in order to protect the rights of the majority. The mood of what was once socially acceptable behavior, is now looked upon as an immoral and degrading habit.

Smoking has clearly, and without a doubt, been linked to at least 30 per cent of all cancer victims. Although cancer and heart disease are listed as America's leading killers, *the biggest underlying cause of death in this country is tobacco use.* A condition that could have been preventable simply through behavioral changes.

Even if you survive a premature demise, smoking may lead to such physical problems as earlier menopause in women, weaker bones, emphysema, and other various diseases. Smoking even compounds those problems of unrelated diseases as well. Arthritis is one such example. Arthritic smokers destroy much of the vitamin C in their body which is necessary for the synthesis of collagen, a critical joint protein.

Perhaps you are one with the attitude, "That the damage has already been done, so why quit now?", listen up! Several years back a group of British researchers study of 18,000 people showed that the ones who smoked for 20 years, but have quit for the last 10, found they had no greater risk of contracting lung cancer than those who had never smoked at all.

Even if you don't care about yourself, it is others around you that also become subjected to the same dangers, says our U.S. Surgeon General, labelling second hand smoke just as toxic and detrimental as taking a puff yourself. And when you finally put all the bits and pieces together and honestly look at the entire picture, one can only conclude that smoking is nothing but vandalistic to health and well-being. A progressive robbing of one's own life-force.

Granted, there will always be those who continue to smoke, but if you still feel you can't kick the habit and quit smoking, you can still benefit more from diet and exercise than those smokers who don't.

DRUGS

It should go without saying that drugs, along with steroids, smoking, and alcohol, have no place anywhere in our world of fitness and health. On this subject, I will not elaborate further, nor should I have to, due to the understanding of basic common sense.

Dare to be different. Stand on your own two feet. Be one above the crowd rather, than trying so hard to be one in it. For it will always be YOUR decision, to JUST SAY NO!

STEP II:

BECOME NUTRITIONALLY SOUND

CHAPTER FOUR:

LET'S EAT!

Physically speaking, our so-called model society of today is, arguably, in the worst state of health in recent history. Despite all of the medical technology, studies and research that has been made available, the average person is still, by many standards, out of shape. Lack of exercise, inadequate eating habits, and a continued recklessness of one's dietary beliefs have, somehow, held on as our primary dilemma.

This chapter is where it all must begin. Your *most direct route* to "getting the look" must always begin here! Contrary to what many still believe, the first step towards genuine fitness begins right at your own dinner table, *before* one ever lifts a single barbell, or jogs that first lap around the block.

To fully grasp today's problems, it helps to be able to first understand the relationship our past has played in the forming of such modern day food fiascoes. A history that has become rich in misuse and taking things for granted.

For history has shown, that our present day eating habits, regardless of body type, have traditionally formed from the labor-oriented lifestyle of our ancestors. Back in a time revered as "the good ol' days", when life was colored as simple and uncomplicated, yet a hard life compared to today's standards. Their average way of life was much more active and required a larger amount of physical exertion, which in turn, justified a larger appetite. (Building cabins, loading trucks, farming, etc.)

But today, with mechanization replacing more and more bona fide manpower, our bodies have become geared much differently than those of yesteryear. For the most part, we have quickly developed into a generation of inactive, ever-consuming softies. To make matters worse, not only we, as the supposed mature and knowledgeable adults, but also our children, continue to indulge the thought of eating anything we want and get away with it. An accumulative, "faster the better, worry about it later" attitude that dramatically veers from the path of basic, good wholesome foods and proper eating practices.

So where lies the fault? Who, or where, can we point the finger? Some blame our forever new and developing space-age technology as the leading culprit. Undeniably, it has made eating much too easy and convenient whether at home or eating out. Frozen "heat and eat" dinners, microwaves, and fast food restaurants have revolutionized the way we prepare and eat our meals. We must admit, by most standards, we, the eating consumer have it pretty easy today compared to those of yesteryear. But unfortunately, many times when you have too much of a good thing, there tends to be a certain amount of abuse. That's right, in this instance, it's FOOD.

Actually, our present day nutritional needs compared to those before us haven't changed all that much, just the manner in which we get them. This translates into terms of not really how much you eat, but more importantly, what you eat and what your body actually needs. That's right, what exactly *does it need?*

BASIC NEEDS

Each of us, whether you are short, tall, skinny or obese, have specific nutritional needs that must be met in order to maintain normal bodily functions. These needs are called your *basic maintenance requirements.* As previously mentioned, these requirements are largely determined by your present and on-going activity levels.

Ask yourself, just how active are you on an average day? And when I say active, I mean <u>physically</u> active. Simply labelling yourself a perpetually busy person, or perhaps one who stands on your feet at work all day just doesn't count.

For example, take a person who works construction for a living. This type of individual will probably have higher nutritional requirements than one who merely sits behind a desk or the wheel of a car. That particular person, behind the wheel and others like them, usually will have a *lower* metabolic rate than that of the other just described. In other words, they will have more of a tendency to burn their food less efficiently, whereby having the potential of creating a nutritional imbalance. From here it's not too hard to see where this can all lead.

Therefore, **there must**, at some point, be an effort to <u>balance</u> what you eat according to how active you are. Enter, the dynamic duo.

THE DYNAMIC DUO

Eating right is one thing, BUT, the fitness puzzle cannot be successfully completed until the remaining piece has been added. That's right, the "E" word. Your dreams of a flat tummy and trim thighs all ride on this final and absolute concept;

PROPER EATING HABITS <u>*along with*</u> PROPER EXERCISE, must be emphasized and executed with **equal** importance.

Just as Batman needs Robin and government needs taxes, it's got to be a 50-50 relationship. Believe it! If you don't, you might as well quit right now, because there is nothing in this world that will replace it. Diet and exercise. Exercise and diet. Any time you decide to split up this combo, YOU *WILL* FAIL, period! I apologize for sounding so blunt, but it's a fundamental equation that has long since passed the tests of time and technology.

I also realize this is probably nothing new, and hearing it again and again gets pretty old, but far too many still believe, or desperately WANT to believe, that as long as they

22

make the attempt to eat right now and then, they can achieve the same results *without exercise.* Wrong! Wrong! Wrong! One cannot go without the other, period!

Believing in this, and truly accepting it, true to heart, will be your first and one of your most important cardinal rules to live by. If not, the battle is already lost.

(I realize that by introducing this 50-50 concept, or mentioning the word *exercise* at this early stage in the middle of a diet chapter may seem awkward and somewhat out of place, but it is a necessary precursor for forming the correct mind-set later on, and yes, you WILL see it again and again.)

THE DREADED WORD

We now come to the old saying "you are what you eat". Frighteningly enough, this can be fairly close to the truth, although it is more to the thought that it pertains to.

However, it is that infamous, little four letter word, that persuades one to either quit or conquer. That word,....... DIET. There, I said it. Don't be afraid and quit on me now, hang in there! It's not as bad as most make it out to be if one merely hangs in there and sticks with the basics. Nevertheless, it will be the main point of focus throughout this particular chapter. (Exercise being the other half is dealt with in later chapters.)

For so many, the word *diet* is at the very least, scary, intimidating, and often associated with failure. It has been largely stereotyped to be this dreaded, sacrifice at-all-cost attitude, which in turn, greatly intimidates those who start, as well as those toying with the idea of changing culinary practices.

I have found this to be especially true because of how the health community inadvertently overly complicates the issue with jillions of articles, weight loss programs, videos, cook books, and numerous statistics. Looking at the big picture all at one time, is and can be, a frightening experience.

There is a dire need for a **simplified** mindset the average person can follow and understand. An approach that leans heavily towards practicality and simple everyday life.

So here it is. The old interpretation of the word *diet* and what it has grown to represent in the past is now gone, erased, extinct. Now is the time to wipe the old slate clean, a time to re-program. From this point on, our true definition and new-way attitude towards the word *diet* is;

DIETING ------> Eating Healthy, Eating for Life!
Nothing more and nothing less.

(Later on in this chapter, I will show you exactly what I mean by revealing a simple, but effective one-two punch approach. However, now is not the time. Please continue.)

DIFFERENT MEANING FOR DIFFERENT PEOPLE

Clearly, your interpretation of what dieting represents does not always carry the same meaning and purpose than it does with others. While most regard diet as a way to lose weight, others view it as a way to gain, or simply to preserve. To a certain degree, this is true, but it is also false.

Webster's dictionary defines diet as, a: food and drink regularly provided, b: habitual nourishment, c: to cause to eat and drink or according to prescribed rules.

It says nothing at all about losing weight, gaining weight, or juggling recipes. There is nothing in it that implies the misconstrued meaning that it still carries today.

Again, the "D" word itself should represent nothing more than a modest lifestyle change to *eating healthier*. It is a modernistic concept that should be taken and used for what it really is.

GOING TO THE EXTREME

Since eating healthier should now be our primary focus, I could not in good conscience, leave out this next pitfall many believe to be their most direct route to dietary success, *fad diets*.

Admittedly, either you or someone you know have probably experienced a certain degree of weight loss success by diligently following many of the popular fad diets that have come along, each one claiming to be *the one*. You know, the ones that seem to take us all by storm, in turn, creating a herd-type mentality. An overwhelming temptation to sit on an already crowded bandwagon of followers. The protein diet, the carbohydrate diet, the complete meal in a drink diet, the appetite suppressing pill, this diet program, that diet program, on and on and on.

Yes, there probably was some measurable degree of weight loss during the initial attempt, or in many cases, attempt*s*. But the true kicker here is, the results are, at best, **short lived**, and involve **going to the extreme**. In short, those fad diets that proscribe eating on either extreme, such as eating *only* foods high in protein, or *only* foods high in carbohydrates, or *only* foods low in fat, and so on.

You know as well as I that too much of any one thing is not good for you. Like everything else, MODERATION and BALANCE is the key. This approach, and this only, will be your most direct route to successful eating. Believe it! (I will show you exactly what I mean a little later.) Extreme dieting is, in most cases, unhealthy, unproductive, definitely uninspiring, and just plain no fun!

Do you really want to go to such extremes by following such fad diets? Do you really want to eat this way for the rest of your life? Are the principles you are following sound and based on something you can stick with day in and day out, forever? Look around you, do the results from these magnificent diets really last, for you, your neighbor, for the other millions like you? The answer is painfully obvious.

Again, the word <u>diet</u> (which to me is short for *deprivation*) just doesn't work in the long run. And for most of us, *it's the long run that really counts!*

NUTRITION AND TEENAGERS

In light of eating for the long haul, *proper nutrition* is probably most important at the pre-teen and teenage group, than that of the older, more mature individual. This is primarily due to the fact that the young body is trying to lay its ground work into building the healthiest body it can.

Also, becoming nutritionally sound at this point in time, further conditions and programs proper eating habits for the youngsters later adult years. Most definitely, an uphill climb by today's standards.

Without this ever-so-needed nutritional background at this early age, the chances are slim, that one will ever be able to entirely catch up later on, no matter how hard one tries.

Adolescent Girls

Of the several million Americans with eating disorders, 90% of them are female, most of whom are teenagers. It is truly unfortunate that every year thousands of these teenage girls try to regulate their weight by fasting or eating bread and water diets.

I should again point out, that dieting the wrong way could very well lead to loss of muscle and body composition. Putting it simply, you could lose your shape and figure, even your life. And for most girls, developing and maintaining their figure is their primary concern.

Therefore, common sense should tell you that it really does not pay to sink to such drastic measures in the effort to lose or regulate weight. Instead, it makes more sense to shape and firm through diet and exercise.

Adolescent Boys

As for young boys, many may require up to 4000 calories a day during this time in their life, especially if they are very active. This may help explain the perpetually hungry state they always seem to be in. Here, the adolescent boy is eating so much, that deficiencies should not be a problem. Usually, it's junk food and inactivity that is the problem.

GAINING WEIGHT?

Unlike the majority of those trying to loose weight, there is a smaller percentage of individuals that carry the concept of dieting in yet another direction. Yes, there are those who actually try to gain weight, usually those of the ectomorphic group, (long thin boned, slightly muscled, low body fat).

Many reasons could account for this condition, take genetics for one. Just as the overweight person has to fight against their body's natural genetic ease of gaining weight, the underweight person has to work harder to keep from being too skinny.

Others include the "high strung", continually active individuals, that often deny themselves the chance to put on any appreciable amount of weight, if not for a better reason, simply as a result of their lifestyle. This active, energetic, body type many times does not eat enough throughout the day to support their high metabolism, thus burning anything extra that may have had the chance to accumulate.

Although this problem is quite different, and at times, often admired by those on the opposite side of the fence, the consequences of sporadic eating habits can be just as detrimental to this group as any other.

OTHER DIET RELATED PROBLEMS

Besides those individuals who have to watch their diet because they are overweight or underweight, there other problems that one should be aware of before jumping into any diet/exercise program. Those who suffer from more specialized problems like diabetes, hypoglycemia, and other metabolic disorders, should consult a nutritionally trained physician.

Sure-fire answers for the likes of these and other specialized dietary dilemmas cannot be adequately resolved in a mere paragraph or two, which is why I have offered no specific answer or forgone conclusion for this particular area. Any time you have a special problem, you see a specialist.

FOOD-WISE FACTS

Lets face it, no one likes to have to watch what they eat, but unfortunately, it is now a fact of life. That's right, becoming more **knowledgeable** on the foods you eat, is and should be, a life long habit. Habits that should be permanently engraved in your lifestyle, just as in getting dressed for work or brushing your teeth.

Although repetitive to some, as most habits generally are, these following paragraphs are significant facts you should hopefully by now, be aware of, understand, and fully accept in regards to eating healthier from now on. Some you may recognize, while some you may not, but all are essential toward providing you with a somewhat condensed dietary foundation from which you must continue to build, regardless of what you already know or believe. Again, it all must start right here!

1)   First and foremost, you must have faith in yourself. You will succeed, period! Believe it...in your mind...your thoughts...and your actions.

Re-program your thought patterns by starting anew, beginning with one's faith, motivation, and pride. You **WILL** do what it takes to achieve your dietary goals. Failure at this point is not permissible. Often it will seem hard, but doing it the right way usually is, *in anything.*

You are someone special and a winner in your own way. Whether this is your first try at a weight loss/maintenance program, or your last desperate attempt, fulfillment will come to those who *believe.*

YOU are no different than those who have found success, so avoid negative thoughts and attitudes of failure from those around you. Do not allow anyone to bring you down. Instead, listen only to those individuals with positive thoughts and direction.

Those that make fun or use excuses are usually lazy, weak-minded, or deeply insecure themselves. You are now beginning a new and healthful lifestyle, and those with pessimistic attitudes can either join you, or be left behind.

"The difference between the impossible and the possible lies in a person's determination". -Tommy Lasorda, former manager of the Los Angeles Dodgers.

2)   From this point forward, take control of your life. Don't let food or other bad habits dictate how you live. Studies have shown that those who maintain a regular diet/exercise program, show a higher degree of all-around independence, and are not as likely to allow life (or food) lead them around by the nose. This particular group of people make their own decisions, whether it be at their job, at play, or home at the dinner table.

3)   In starting any kind of new program, whether it be exercise, finance, weight-loss, or job related, you need to have something more than just willpower to get you there. You will have much greater success if you set goals, schedules, and commitments. Just something in concrete form.

And just as important, each of these should be taken in little steps, ones that you are reasonably sure of accomplishing. I say again, little steps. Over time, all those little steps added together will eventually lead you to your final goal. Try it, it really works!

4)   In addition to step progression, learn to use self visualization tactics before your willpower runs out and you end up quitting completely. In other words, *mentally* visualize yourself the way you want to be, then work to get there.

But keep in mind, your final goal destination should never be limited to exact pounds gained or lost, or through constant mirror-checking rituals. There's much more to it than that. The true accomplishments come more from how you **feel on the inside**, as well as sharpening your outward attributes.

5)   If you are the type of person who thinks you can break all the proper nutritional rules and get by with it, think again. Although you presently show no sign, you may find damage or experience health problems later on in your lifetime.

One doesn't have to look very far for proof, either. Of this country's top ten leading causes of death, five are diet-related to some degree. (Cancer, heart disease, stroke, diabetes, and chronic liver disease/cirrhosis.)

So start eating properly now and not wait until it's too late. For if you think about it, *the future of your health has just been determined by what you ate yesterday.*

6)   Now is as good a time as any for you to increase your overall knowledge base on proper nutrition. I like to simply refer to it as getting *food-smart.*

This can be attained through more diverse, food-oriented forms of reading, and being more open to various health related articles, and/or consulting the advice of a qualified nutritionist. These sources of information can be very helpful in starting, assessing, and regulating the perfect diet for you or someone requiring outside assistance.

Again, seek only that help that is reputable. Be aware of so called "counselors", who are really sales-people. Even though they may be trained in such areas as nutrition and weight loss, their efforts seem to be somewhat limited due to the conflict of interest in making that all important buck.

Over time, you should learn to be completely self-sufficient when it comes to all diet matters. Remember, *no one can do it for you.* Why be like so many and pay good money to someone, some product, or some service, for them to turn right around and tell you something you already know, quite simply, eat right and exercise? (Sound familiar?)

LEARN TO FADE-OUT ON THE DEPENDENCY OF OTHERS AND OTHER SUCH DIET RELATED SERVICES AND PROGRAMS, INSTEAD, REPLACING YOUR OWN MIND AS THE POWER SOURCE AND MEANS OF MOTIVATION.

Your body will not only reap wonders from the dietary benefits, but at the same time, you are likely to rediscover such well-rounded qualities as independence and self-sufficiency. Admirable traits well worth striving.

7)   Beware of fads, gimmicks, or promises of overnight results. There is no safe or reputable get-trim-quick solution. This way of thinking is popular with those that

are immature and desperate.

Don't think you can lay on your back, be shaken by some machine and watch the fat disappear and muscle pop out. There are no *magic* pills, potions, programs, or procedures that will make you look like Joe Bodybuilder or Miss Supermodel U.S.A. There is no shortcut or sales pitch that will replace, nor come close to, good old fashion work ethics and <u>honest</u> effort.

8) Never confuse fasting and dieting as the same. *Fasting* your body to lose that unwanted weight quickly can be more harmful and stressful than being overweight. Fasting starves your body of essential nutrients putting it into more of a starvation mode, eventually destroying what health you have left.

In truth, the weight you lose by fasting can be quite misleading, and is usually in the form of water and muscle tissue, *NOT FAT*. Believe it or not, you will experience greater fat loss by eating periodically and exercising, than during starvation.

9) In relation to what was just mentioned, never confine your thoughts of dieting to just bread, water, and rabbit food when you do eat. If you do, your body will again suffer in one way or another. Always remember, an overweight person has the <u>same</u> basic nutritional requirements as one who is more healthy.

The same thing goes with calorie restriction **ONLY** programs. They too, are regarded as crash course programs resulting in failure and poor health. They usually involve some sort of nutrient deprivation, which makes them unsafe and unsuccessful in the long run. Instead, go with those that teach you to eat *healthier*, with the incorporation of exercise.

10) Just as in exercise, your body thrives on the *consistency* of its meals. It responds best when it knows when each meal is coming. Therefore, it is important to remember to spread your eating throughout the day in the form of smaller, consistent meals, rather than gorging on just one large meal.

It has been widely accepted that eating in just such a way, allows your body to do a much better job of digesting and absorbing its food (providing it is done in moderation and consisting of something out of the five basic food groups). Preferably, try to get in **at least** the basic 3 meals per day; breakfast, a noon lunch, and dinner. (Better yet, a small nutritious snack between each.)

Those individuals who believe saving up calories for the indulgence of just one particular meal a day should now know that this so-called "now I can eat as much as I want" approach, is not only unhealthy and tends to throw off their body's normal eating clock, but eventually leads them to overeating and failure in diet in the long run.

29

11) If you feel the need to snack or nibble, or perhaps frequently categorize yourself as an "impulse eater", teach yourself to get into the habit of eating more healthful snacks instead of the traditional junk like cookies, candy or chips. I suggest pick-me-ups, like fresh fruits or low fat granola bars. They will help suppress hunger pangs, along with added nutritional value.

Healthful snacking in this way ensures one rarely gets too hungry. So, when you do finally sit down at the dinner table, you will find yourself less likely to overindulge.

12) A booming problem with most of today's supposed *weight loss/diet programs*, is the tendency to gain back the weight you lost as soon as you leave that diet or program. A good example would be some of our famous television celebrities. One moment they are headline news after losing a considerable amount of weight, often accompanied with a release of their new diet program. Then, a short while later you see them again, after gaining it all back. They, like many of us today, constantly battle to keep off the weight they worked so hard to get rid of.

Why? Because much of it all goes back to how the exercise aspect has been left out, or at least, not emphasized enough. I know, here I go again, but proper *exercise* must go hand in hand with proper *dieting* in order to properly train the body to continue burning fat efficiently. (For more on the how's and why's, see the chapter called "Aerobically Speaking".)

13) Although the diet/exercise theme is continually encouraged everywhere you look, you should still know that there is a proper time and place for everything. A time that the body not only works better, but works safer. That is why you should never eat right before or immediately after each exercise period. The rule to go by is to eat **no sooner** than 1 1/2 hours before or 1 hour after exercise.

During the digestion process, the body focuses its full attention to breaking down and dispersing food for energy. To physically exert yourself at this time not only deprives those muscles you would be exercising of needed energy and oxygen, but significantly increases the amount of stress on the circulatory and respiratory systems respectively.

14) It would be a good idea to have your cholesterol count checked and know where it should be. Although the procedure is simple, there are, oftentimes, variables that must be taken into account in order to achieve any certain degree of accuracy. Having a quick cholesterol count at your local mall or shopping center is not good enough. Therefore, it is recommended that the count be done only by your doctor.

Generally, you want that count to be below 200, with 200 to 230 borderline.

15) Cholesterol is an important thing to keep an eye on, but cutting down on the FAT in your diet should be your main concern. That's right, we've all heard it again and again, day in and day out. It's the saturated fats in the food you eat, more than the cholesterol that becomes the real problem.

As you may know, much of the cholesterol is produced by your own liver. Eating foods high in saturated fats sends the liver a signal to make more cholesterol. Quite simply, fat and cholesterol usually go hand in hand. One more time, "fat and cholesterol go hand in hand".

By knowing and understanding this relationship, it only makes good sense that being more aware of your fat intake will also greatly effect your level of blood cholesterol.

16) Many times, changes in diet do not have to be drastic, just used with a little more common sense. I am referring to substituting high-fat ingredients with those of low-fat equivalents.

For example, you could substitute skim or 2% milk for whole milk, pure vegetable oils for shortening, egg whites for whole eggs, nonfat yogurt for sour cream, lean and select cuts of beef rather than ones higher in fat.

High fat foods are packed full of calories and take a longer time for the body to digest. By simply cutting down, *but not necessarily cutting out*, on such little culinary practices here and there, can, and will, make a considerable difference over a short period of time.

17) Since you will be trying to cut more fatty foods out of your diet, you will no doubt experience some kind of void in your appetite where the fat used to be. A luring emptiness that needs filled, yet, hopefully, one that will quench the appetite in a more productive manner.

That alternative; increase the amount of fiber in your diet plan. "Dietary Fiber" is a large group of foods derived mostly from plant origin, rather than that of animal origin. Such examples include bran, beans, fruits, and vegetables.

The concept and claims of high fiber diets are well known and fairly undisputed. Present and ongoing research indicates high fiber diets deter various cancer causing diseases, heart disease, high blood cholesterol, and greatly aids those with symptoms of diabetes. These are just a few among a wide range of other healthful benefits.

What many like most is that a high fiber diet can actually help control weight. The reasoning here is two-fold; One, is that more of the high fat foods have been replaced with that of high fiber alternatives. The other, is the way high diets disallow the body from absorbing fat as efficiently as it would have otherwise fiber.

Although increasing one's dietary fiber is a must, one should also recognize it as a gradual process. Never begin too quickly by bulking out on the stuff, thinking the more the better. Instead, allow your body time to adapt to this new way of eating, just as in starting anything new and different.

18) I am a firm believer in that no one gets something worthwhile without some kind of sacrifice. A nutritionally sound body is one of these. My three brothers and I seem to be a prime example of what proper nutrition on a long term basis will yield. It is now easy to look back and appreciate the true devotion our parents made in making sure we always had *good* food on the table.

Many times while we were growing up, my parents sacrificed many of life's little extras and what spare money they did have for good, basic, wholesome food (sometimes whether we liked it or not). Rarely were they the quick and easy, heat and eat dinners, but rather complete and fully prepared meals. This was unlike many of my boyhood friends whose mothers did just enough to get by. They did less actual cooking, instead, feeding their families TV dinners, pizza, fast food, etc.

The point I am trying to make is that all four of us were, and still to this day, are very active physically. We can always be found in any one of a variety of organized sports, or simply enjoying such outdoor activities like motorcycling, fishing, or hunting. Up through the years, and now as adults, not one of us has had any serious medical problems, injuries, or broken bones.

Trust me! I've been through everything from football to Karate, and can honestly say, my body has been severely tested. I have been in quite a few SERIOUS crashes in my pole vaulting years that could have killed me, or at the very least, should have broken some bones. It's as if my bones seem to be superior in strength and elasticity, compared to those of my friends and competitors, who were always breaking something. Again, I must give the credit to my nutritional upbringing. Thanks Mom and Dad! It was worth it.

19) Last but not least, life is meant to be enjoyed. And eating is part of that enjoyment. You will find your body to be very forgiving in what you put into it.

I seem to be a good example of this. From my teenage years up through the present, I still enjoy cakes, cookies, and lots of ice cream. But I want to point out that these "forbidden fruits" are only a small part of my daily diet plan, making them the exception and not the rule.

After all, we are all only human. Each of us it seems, carries an inevitable weakness when it comes to certain foods. Consequently, each of us must make a continued effort towards educating oneself on nutritional matters, and make eating, once again, one of life's simple pleasures.

Remember, *nutrition does not necessarily have to be perfect, just reasonable.*

**************** Stay With Me ***************

Are you still with me? Don't quit on me now. More importantly, don't quit on yourself. Believe it or not, everything mentioned is still part of *the most direct route* concept. Up to this point, you nearly have most of what you will need to know in regard to how you will eat from now on. But before I reveal the final one-two punch approach to eating, you must first re-learn the nutritional basics. So stay with me and hang in there just a little longer. You are almost there. *Almost!*

****

BACK TO THE BASICS - A TRUE BALANCING ACT!

Far to many of you still continue to downplay the importance of true *balance* in the daily diet and what it can do for you and your physical goals. Yea, Yea, you've heard it before. But really think about this word, "balance". Balance plays a key role in all aspects of life such as in religion, relationships, work, play, and yes, diet.

Balance - Without it, few positive changes can ever take place. With it, comes health, happiness, and prosperity.

Therefore, to ensure you are selecting the proper foods for that body you are taking care of so well, YOU MUST, include something from each of the five main food groups below each and <u>every day</u>. (Actually, there are six distinct food groups, but for dietary reasons we will only be concerned with five, leaving out the Fats, Oils, and Sweets group.)
I say again, include something from EACH of the bottom five food groups, EACH AND EVERY DAY!

Group I   ---->   Milk, Yogurt, & Cheese
Group II   ---->   Meat, Poultry, Fish, Dry Beans, Eggs, & Nuts
Group III ---->   Vegeatables
Group IV ---->   Fruits
Group V   ---->   Bread, Cereal, Rice, & Pasta

(not necessarily listed in order of importance)

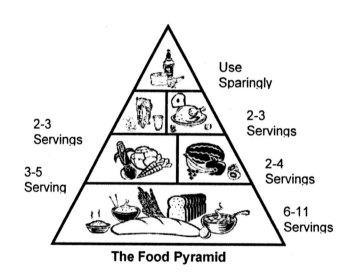

The Food Pyramid

This is simply an updated version from the long-time standby of the *basic four* of years past. This graphic, resembling a pyramid, has now been accepted as the basis for the ideal diet as determined by the U.S. Department of Agriculture.

The reasoning behind the design is simple; to make it easier for the eating consumer to understand what foods they need, from which group, and in what amounts.

Preferably, one should make up a greater portion of their diet from those foods that make up the larger base (grains), compared to those nearer the top as the pyramid narrows (fats and oils). Quite simply, eat lots from the bottom, some from the middle, and just a teeny bit off the top. Regardless, each group of foods have their place in our daily regimen with one just as important as the other, the only exception is the *amount required.*

The following is a breakdown of what is contained in the food pyramid. Although you may already be familiar with or have seen the given information listed before, again, I feel it is important enough to re-emphasize and include it in this chapter.

We begin by listing the four basic elements needed for normal bodily functions; water, fats, proteins, and carbohydrates.

Water

Often not regarded as a nutritional necessity, water should be just as much a part of the diet as the foods you eat. Actually, water should be considered your *main nutrient.*

Water functions in cleansing the internal organs, flushing out toxins, thins the blood, and cools the body after a workout. It aids in the recovery of both muscle and the brain, and can also be used as an appetite suppressor. Drinking adequate amounts of water also lubricates your skin, giving it that young and healthy look.

You should drink *at a minimum* 2-3 glasses per day, or one glass per meal, **not including** beverages such as soft drinks, coffee, etc. And for those with problems of water retention, simply avoid those diets high in sodium.

I say again and take this as serious as a heart attack, *drink water and lots of it.* That means especially before, during, and after your workout.

Keeping your body sufficiently hydrated will do wonders for your body and soul along with many far-reaching effects most are probably not aware of (losing fat, lowering blood pressure, stress, etc.) For more on this I strongly recommend you find time to read "Your Body's Many Cries For Water", by F. Batmanghelidj, M.D.

Fats

Yes, you may not think so, but fats *are* important in your diet. They play an essential role in providing energy for muscle use. Aside from being the greatest source of energy for the human body, fat also functions to lubricate your body parts, aids in the carrying of certain vitamins, and provides heating of the body itself.

Unfortunately for most of us, it is many of these same fats in our foods that tempt and stimulate our taste buds to eat the way we do. Fat adds flavor and a sort of zeal that sparks the palate and enhances the enjoyment of eating.

But for the most part, you shouldn't have to worry about not getting enough fat in your diet. With the foods we eat today, it would be almost impossible not to get the necessary recommended allowance of fat. The obvious problem is getting too much.

Protein

In the muscle building process, the importance of protein in your diet cannot be stressed enough. This important element is essential for muscle maintenance, repair, and growth. Choosing a good protein source should be in the form of lean or low-fat meats, such as fish and poultry. Combination dishes like beans and rice also work well. Dried beans, lentils, and split peas are even lower in fats and make them an excellent meat substitute.

Carbohydrates

In order to utilize the available protein in your current diet, you must also have a good balance of carbohydrates. They fuel your system by raising the blood sugar level, thus providing the muscle with energy. You can find carbohydrates in cereal grains, breads, pastas, and also in roughage's like fruits and vegetables. Again, most of your diet should consist of foods derived from this particular group.

Vitamins and Minerals

Proper nutrition is never complete without vitamins and minerals. Preferably, we should get these vitamins and minerals from the food we eat, <u>through our three or more daily balanced meals.</u>

Vitamin A: (dark, leafy greens, milk, especially fortified milk, eggs, spinach, carrots, liver, broccoli, sweet potatoes as well as all other deep yellow vegetables and fruits) Promotes good vision as well as skin texture.

Vitamin B: (fish, whole grains, wheat germ, poultry, milk, fruit, eggs, liver, beans, and green vegetables) Promotes proper functioning of nervous system, digestive tract, mental alertness, preservation of muscle, and aids in protection against infections.

Vitamin C: (citrus fruits, dark, leafy greens, vegetables, tomato's, potatoes, berries, honeydew) Aids in the body's ability to resist infection, aiding in the healing process, while strengthening vascular and skeletal systems. Vitamin C is also involved in the production of connective tissue, iron absorption, and collagen formation.

Vitamin D: (direct sunlight, milk, eggs, chicken livers, fish) Very important in promoting strong bones and teeth. You should know your skin manufactures it's own Vitamin D but needs ultra violet rays from the sun to get it started. It only takes around 15 minutes per day on hands and face to get what is recommended.

Vitamin E: (dark, leafy green vegetables and vegetable oils, eggs, whole grains, and wheat germ) Aids in the normal function of the circulatory system, also contributing to the respiratory and reproductive systems respectively.

Minerals: (whole grains, lean meat, fish, legumes, deep green vegetables) The body also requires certain quantities of minerals, that work with vitamins towards promoting total body health. They are just as important as vitamins, even though required in smaller amounts. Calcium, phosphorus, iron, magnesium, iodine, zinc, sodium, copper, potassium, and manganese.

Again, these essential nutrients can all be properly acquired by including something from each of the five basic food groups every day. It couldn't be any simpler.

Every other day or so, check to make sure no one food group has been left out or neglected. If it was, INCLUDE it! As the saying goes, "JUST DO IT!"

VITAMIN SUPPLEMENTATION

Never rely on vitamins or other methods of supplementation, for the purpose of REPLACING good food and healthy eating habits.

It's no secret to anyone that the use of vitamins and other related food supplements has become ever-increasingly big business, in turn, bringing all kinds of promises, charts, and statistics of what adding vitamins to your diet can do for you. As a result, we have become bombarded with all sorts of gimmicks and bogus brand name vitamin and vitamin off-shoots, thus, leaving us with the feeling that we can't live right without them. It can become very confusing and quite expensive.

This, along with the wide range of potential health problems associated with this topic, is why individual solutions cannot be properly addressed here in book form. There are just too many factors to consider. Some examples include pregnant women, the elderly in a retirement home, a woman on a strict diet program, and clearly, the professional athlete. All of which may be susceptible to various vitamin deficiencies due to exceptional conditions.

If this pertains to you, most find that taking a multi-vitamin will provide a little added insurance. Always check the label to ensure that 50-150% of U.S. Recommended Daily Allowance is provided.

But for most of us, spending money on vitamins and other food supplements, for, shall we say, "insurance reasons", is generally unnecessary. *You can get everything your body needs just by making sure you don't skip any one of the five food groups every day. It is as simple as that.* Just eat right and spend your money on cuisine your body actually needs.

FAT B GONE - PUNCH #1

All right now, it's time for the one-two punch I promised you. With the dietary foundation now in place, I will, at this point, attempt to guide you in a simple, uncomplicated manner that will allow you to finally regain control over your dietary health in a manner that is sensible and effective. Punch #1 goes something like this:

IT'S NOT NECESSARILY HOW MUCH YOU EAT THAT REALLY COUNTS, BUT RATHER, HOW MUCH OF **WHAT** *YOU EAT!*

If you guessed too much fat as the primary focus here, congratulations, you're right on. But you probably already knew that, didn't you? Well, too bad! Because from now on, each and every one of you, regardless of whether or not you fit in the overweight or borderline category, MUST get into the daily habit of reading food labels (*Nutrition Facts*) and tracking your *FAT CONTENT* on a per serving basis (The Total amount of fat in each Tbsp., tsp., 1/2 cup, 1 slice, etc.) I realize this seems troublesome and a bit of a hassle, but there must be no more guessing or looking for ways around it, just do it! **You must know just exactly where the fat in your diet is coming from.**

This particular method of tracking fat intake will leave you with a much broader perspective as to not only where the problem lies, but what it's going to take for you to correct it. (Trust me, it's here where your blurred picture of past dietary practices will soon come into focus.)

Remember, keep believing in yourself. Do not accept failure before first giving yourself a chance to succeed. Don't make this appear to be any harder than what it is, because it's not. This will be just like anything else in your life, *what you make of it!*

For your convenience, I have provided much of what you will need to track your *food fat* towards the back of this book in the section called, "Food Reference Guide". Here, you will find a complete listing of almost every food out there, similar in a way to other such volumes of information, EXCEPT this listing deals only with fat gram content, leaving out all the rest of the mind-boggling numbers and statistics regarding nutrient value. As an added bonus, the calorie content of each food is also provided for those die-hard calorie counters who know of no other way with which to monitor their food intake.

*********** Calorie Counting - yes or no? ***********

Counting and tracking one's caloric intake is also very important to know exactly where you need to make your dietary stand. Federal guidelines state that the average consumer get no more than 30% of their calories from fat.

But the reason I stray from the using a calorie approach is because if you give the average consumer a choice between eating an apple with 125 calories and a Devils Food Snack Cake with 105 calories, they will usually choose the latter. Simply stated, don't completely ignore caloric content, instead, pay more attention to the source of *where* the calories came from, rather than number *totals*.

****

One more little hint of advice; I further recommend the purchase of a pocket-sized, smaller version food listing. They are relatively inexpensive and can be found in just about any nutrition store. They are compact in size, thus making them a readily available tool when grocery shopping, eating out, and so on. The next step up and a little more on the elaborate side, is the opportunity to select from a variety of home computer software or internet related web sites that make it easier than ever to track and automatically calculate such information for you. It's your choice. Choose it, then use it!

PUNCH #2 - THE KNOCKOUT

And finally, a simple, yet self-sufficient, one answer approach to eating right. No curves, no multi-leveled paths to take, no brain-busting terminology, and no beating around the bush. Just results!

Start by simply consulting the food listing provided in the back of the book, then add up the number of total fat grams in each of the foods you eat on a day by day basis. At the end of the day, the total should fall on, or somewhere between;

30-60 g/day for the average male
30-50 g/day for the average female.

No more and no less, (except for extenuating circumstances). Pretty easy, huh? If you find yourself out of the given range either way, get back in it! Especially if you are consuming anything over 60 grams of fat per day.

***************** Wean yourself *****************

But use caution and take it slow. Here, long-term success will largely be determined by how gradually you make the cuts. In other words, if you are well over the limit, DON'T immediately cut back to 50 or 60 grams the first day or even the first week. Preferably, try not to cut more than a total of 10 grams of dietary fat at any one time, instead, spread the cut-back process out over a couple of weeks or more. Remember, we are cutting down, *not cutting out!*

****

Believe it or not, this approach allows you to eat every meal until you are satisfied, as long as most of the higher fat foods have been substituted with more healthy choices. Just think, no more counting calories. No more deprivation. No more figuring percentages. No more continued frustration and self-doubt. Those who want to lose the fat for good can now get it done. Others striving to gain quality weight or simply trying to maintain, will now know where they stand nutritionally versus where they need to be.

I would be remiss if I failed to give due credit to the one who first came up with this approach. His name is Dr. Martin Katahn, Professor of psychology and director of the Vanderbilt Weight Management Program at Vanderbilt University. He authored a former #1 best seller over ten years ago, among a handful of other diet-related works, to his name. Although his concept is a little dated doesn't mean it won't work in today's world. Many times you have to look *backward* to find what really works over the long haul. Surprisingly, I have found that some of the best concepts in health and fitness are like buried treasures, just waiting for someone to stumble upon them.

Originally, Dr. Katahn's fat gram approach was a little on the strict side of the bottom end, however, the Food and Drug Administration recently revealed that everyone, regardless of condition, requires at least 30 grams of fat per day for normal bodily functions. In contrast, The American Heart Association gives a top end limit of 80 fat grams per day. So, with these figures as our starting point and after juggling the numbers here and there, you and I now have a target range in which to shoot for.

EXAMPLE #1

This represents an average diet on an average day. Note how this is well within the accepted range of daily fat grams for an average male and where not all fat has been removed, just cut to a more reasonable level. Also notice that there is something included from each of the basic food groups, spread *evenly* throughout the day. It's not overly lenient, yet none too strict.

		fat grams
breakfast	plain corn flakes	
	w/ 2% milk	5
	orange juice	0
	toast w/ 1pat butter	5
snack	banana	0
	chocolate chip cookie	3
lunch	turkey ham sandwich	
	w/ fresh spinach leaves	18
	ice water	0
	plain corn chips	5
	apple	0
snack	granola bar	5
	canned peaches	0
dinner	2.5 oz lean, broiled	
	sirloin steak	6
	Baked potato w/1 pat	
	butter, 1 Tbsp sour cream	7
	green beans	0
	canned pears	0
	french bread	1
	ice water or tea	0
snack	chocolate	1
	frozen yogurt	
		56 fat grams

41

Now notice example #2. This particular diet of the day contains too much fat and not enough balance of breads, fruits, and vegetables. Here, a *gradual*, but deliberate cut back on fat is needed, in turn, replacing it with more of those foods that make up the bottom half of the food pyramid.

Example #3 is almost as bad. This represents a diet many still believe to be acceptable. Remember, you cannot save up fat grams or calories in hopes of being able to tank up on just one particular meal a day. Even though this example is still within the daily fat gram range, this method of eating will do more harm to the body than good.

WRONG!
EXAMPLE #2

			WRONG! EXAMPLE #3	
2 eggs	12	**breakfast**	coffee	0
2 sausage strips	7		1 doughnut	6
hash browns	12			
biscuits & gravy	2			
coffee	0			
candy bar	12	**snack**	4 saltine crackers	1
chefs salad w/ low-cal. dressing	30	**lunch**	side salad w/ low-cal dressing	2
soft drink	0		soft drink	0
sm ice cream cone	4			
1 bag of M&M choco-coated peanuts	12	**snack**	hard candy	0
3 oz. reg cut roast	24	**dinner**	1 reg cut pork chop	21
potatoes & gravy	4		baked potato w/ 1	
dinner roll	3		Tbsp sour cream & butter	5
green beans	0		whole kernel corn	0
iced tea	0		Lg buttered dinner roll	10
			ice tea	0
2 chocolate chip cookies	6		apple pie	15
	128 fat grams			**60 fat grams**

Do yourself a favor and pay close attention to the actual serving size of each of your food portions when adding it all up. Honestly ask yourself, did you spoon in a cup of your favorite ice cream, or was it more like four times that amount?

And finally, after a couple of months reading food labels, keeping track of fat grams, and in general, acquiring a certain "food sense", you will probably find that recognizing and selecting the right foods will be more automatic, rather than an effort. In short, *no more counting anything*! When this happens, you're well on your way.

THE PERFECT DIET?

In closing this particular chapter, one should now have a pretty good idea on what to expect from oneself from an eating standpoint. Up to this point, the principals of proper eating should be fairly cut and dried with few in-betweens.

Yet, many of you will continue to frantically search for that guaranteed 100% perfect diet. A no-brainer that requires no effort. And why not? You would think that during this scientific day and age with all that we already know on top of what we continue to learn every day, one should be able to reach right out and grasp that one, majestic, "Holy Grail" of diet programs that would ultimately befit us all. A singular, yet simple source for eminent success, regardless of specifics.

Realistically, is there such a thing? Could it ever really be possible? Is there anything out there than can flat guarantee each and every one of us dietary success?

To put it in a nutshell, NO! There is no, *ONE, ABSOLUTE* diet that will ultimately work for everyone. Not this book, that book, or any other book or program. There are simply too many variables to consider, each one ever-changing on an individual basis. In short, everyone is different, in their make-up, mannerisms, and lifestyle. So where does one turn if all else fails?

Not surprisingly, the answer is within you. That's right! It is *your own body* that becomes the key to everlasting dietary success. Your body is the ultimate in supreme knowledge when it comes to taking care of <u>you</u>. Up to now, taking the body for granted and leaning on others for answers has always been and continues to be our biggest downfall.

Therefore, we must all take the initiative to re-learn to tap in and listen, to your bodies needs and wants. More importantly, learn to distinguish between the two. For if you demand a little more effort from yourself, rather than leaning too heavily on others, the results and feedback you encounter will be rewarded tenfold. And NOW is as good a time as any to start.

MORE FOOD FOR THOUGHT

- Fresh foods are generally better than ones that are frozen.
  Frozen foods are generally better than ones that are canned.
  Raw foods are generally better than ones that are cooked.
  Broiled foods are generally better than ones that are fried.
  Steamed foods are generally better than ones that are boiled.

- Begin cautiously when starting any diet/exercise program.

- A diet should never be considered a punishment, but rather a mere fact of life. It is a lifelong quest that requires the same attention, energy, and input, as you would in your job, relationship, etc.

- **Dieting alone** will not firm, shape, or create muscles.

- In the beginning, dieting by itself may allow you to lose a little weight, but in the long run, IT WILL NOT KEEP IT OFF! And that's what really counts!

- Active, dieting women should be concerned with getting their required, crucial nutrients, whereas men need to be on the lookout for more excesses.

- Those who categorize themselves as vitamin worshipers should modify their supplemental agenda by learning to shop more from the greengrocer, instead of a pharmacy.

- Drink plenty of water. It contains zero calories and is a basic necessity for normal bodily functions.

- Eat your meals slowly, preferably, not in less than 20 minutes.

- Avoid going longer than 5 hours without eating.

- *Plan* your dinner meals. Avoid "winging it".

- Keep your mealtime interesting by trying at least one new healthful recipe every month.

- There is nothing wrong with keeping some ready-to-eat snacks in your desk drawer at work, or lunch box in the car in the event you miss lunch, as long as they are nutritious.

- Pack more nutritious lunches from home, rather than *packing it on* via your favorite noon-time eat-outs.

- Avoid eating when bored. If you have a hard time deciding what to eat, you are probably not hungry.

- Avoid eating too much of the processed foods. They often contain too much fat and salt.

- If you tell yourself, "I'll hate myself in the morning for eating this," trust me, you probably will.

- Purchase a fat and/or calorie counter, one small enough to fit in your pocket.

- Keep it simple. Concern yourself more with cutting out on foods that are predominantly high in saturated fats. By doing so, you will not only decrease consumption of fats, but also that of excess cholesterol, sodium, and many unwanted calories.

- Typically, if you make a *consistent*, dedicated effort towards eating lower-fat foods, sooner or later you'll begin to perfer foods that are low in fat.

- Keep abreast on new developments in health-oriented menus provided by your favorite restaurant or other various eating establishments. Times change, and so does eating out.

- Using a worst case scenario.......... Even if you don't watch your diet as close as you should, just being *more aware* of what you do eat along with reading food labels and such, is a definite step in the right direction. Often, this new-found state of awareness leads to the shocking realization of all of the junk, additives and by-products that have been habitually consumed for years. Yuck!

- **The dependency upon diet programs and other related products and services are only part of the solution. The real heart of the matter to eating properly and getting fit, actually lies within <u>oneself.</u>**

- Pay more attention to what your mirror tells you, rather than focusing entirely upon your bathroom scales. Mirrors never lie!

- If you're one of those fortunate enough to be in good shape at this particular point, for you, <u>prevention</u> will be the key. Quite simply, **don't get fat!** And if you have kids, **don't let your kids get fat!**

- Finally, listen to your conscience, for it will further help in guiding you. Deep down inside, you most likely know what is good for you and what isn't. The question is, will you do what it takes? Will you?

STEP III:

EXERCISE, JUST SAY YES!

Whoa, not so fast! As promised, I want you to know that you are almost there. But before you enter into this or any other exercise program, there are certain thoughts and principals that again, must first be acknowledged and understood before undergoing such activity. The ones that require you to <u>think</u> first, long before the first "uumpph" is ever uttered.

Therefore, these next couple of chapters are designed to more easily *lead* you into the following fitness program, thus providing an indication of not only what to expect, but what is expected.

****

CHAPTER FIVE:

USE YOUR HEAD

Unfortunately, the concept of exercise and weight control has long been associated with physical exertion ONLY. With a huff here and a puff there, many still neglect the importance of using the POWER OF THE MIND and the results it can play in an exercise program. Whether you are into weight training, aerobics, or both, this will probably be THE most important concept one can learn from this book.

NOW IS THE TIME TO BEGIN WORKING **SMARTER**, NOT NECESSARILY HARDER!

Because now, more than ever, it has become increasingly easier to differentiate between those who focus *only* on going through the *physical* motions of exercise, compared to those more successful, who are able to include and utilize their own, self-guided, mental powers. Without doubt, those individuals who are able to use the mind effectively, will physically leave behind their counterparts who simply go through the motions.

Don't misunderstand me, going through the motions of exercise is better than not exercising at all. However, the results become frustratingly few and far between. Just as in the previous chapter about reshaping our eating habits, we must also learn and teach ourselves to exercise SMART. In other words, learning to do it right the first time and cut out on all wasted, or perhaps in other terms, non-resulting efforts.

Especially for beginners. The ability to get off on the right foot most often determines the difference between success or failure in the long run.

Likewise, for the more exercise experienced, especially those involved in weight training. Here, one should honestly question whether or not he or she is getting all of what is possible out of what's presently being done.

Just ask yourself, how many times has it been that your only accomplishment was breaking a little sweat, burning a few calories, and providing your conscious with a somewhat contented feeling of finishing another workout? That's all. How long has it been since you've actually seen any concrete evidence of noticeable improvement toward your pre-set goals? Unfortunately, and to the dismay of so many, one eventually comes to learn that their past or present routines have proven just not good enough.

Well, now is the time to change all that. From this point forward you will maximize the results for each and every minute you put into each and every workout, through *mental concentration*. That's right, using your head in conjunction with your body.

Without concentration, nothing can be achieved, with it, anything can be achieved.

I cannot stress this concept enough. It is essential that you master your conscious thoughts and form that critical, *mind-body link*. You must THINK about each and every rep, of each and every exercise. You must THINK about that muscle you are trying to build and tone, and then *mentally* crawl into it, linking it with your mind. FEEL the stretch, FEEL the contraction. CONCENTRATE on, and ISOLATE only, that particular muscle or muscle group you are working, nothing else!

The same goes with aerobic-type exercises as well. Reach deep, learn to re-experience such things as your newly arising metabolic rate, vigor, and vitality. Welcome such often-time forgotten feelings of increased blood flow and overall muscle stimulation. FEEL, DECIPHER, and ANALYZE just what is going on inside, as well as what is transforming on the outside. MENTALLY experience the warmth and satisfaction that exercise provides.

This is what I refer to as the "meat" of our exercise sandwich. Therefore, from this point forward, you must work a little each day towards THINKing yourself healthy. The balance of mind and exercise (especially weight training) should be approached the same as the diet/exercise relationship, that of 50-50. You should now know that only through devoted concentration will you be able to achieve quicker, more long lasting results.

But be advised, this new way of thinking may not come easy at first to all who try it. More often than not, it will require various levels of persistence, dedication, and a great deal of patience. Some will pick up on it faster while others may feel a bit of a struggle. In either case, it WILL come to those who put forth the effort.

Rest assured, I will be with you every step of the way, continually pounding this into your head. Learn to *use your head*! It is just that important!

WANT AND DESIRE

Do you have what it takes to gain the necessary steps toward achieving your physical goals? Obviously you've got an interest, or you wouldn't be reading this now. This is where your level of WANT and DESIRE come in.

Just how bad do you want it?

How badly do you want to trim those thighs or tighten that stomach? How badly do you want that look and feel of total fitness?

Ultimately, it will all come down to your inner WANT and DESIRE! A fit body can be acquired by almost anyone, but unfortunately, many lack the drive and self discipline needed to carry them through. It has to come *from you, for you*, and no one else. Not from your coach, parents, spouse, boyfriend or girlfriend. For without that inner drive or self motivation, it will be hard to maintain dedication to your cause.

Although different levels of *want* and *desire* are present in each and every one of us, no one but you, as an individual, has the last say in determining your physical limits. No one!

PRIORITIES

The same thing also holds true here. If you want anything bad enough, whether it be physically fit or in a certain income bracket for example, you WILL in some way, do what it takes to get it done.

Picture this, throughout our past, man's dire need for food was deemed #1 priority. Therefore, man needs food, man does what it takes to get food, even to the point of killing for it. And now, at present, if man wants a new ski boat for example, man finds some way to budget his income to get it, even if it means sacrificing things he deems more important (paying bills on time, new shoes for Billy, spending more time at work than with family, etc.) Somehow, someway, one way or another, he gets his boat.

Now do this: look around and take notice of everything you have, whether it be a little or a lot, material or immaterial, spiritual or otherwise. What you will find, is that everything you have acquired is EXACTLY what you have wanted. No more and no less. All are concrete, or at best, subtle reminders of what you have fought, sweat, bargained, or continuously worked for.

Now then, look around at what you don't have. A new car, better financial situation, better health or spiritual well-being, whatever it is, it was probably pushed too far down on your things-to-do list. With this simple proof of where you stand at the moment, WHY then can you not achieve complete fitness through better eating and a little exercise?

Why? Because it all comes down to another important concept I want to plant into your mind, and that is, the setting of your *priorities*.

Granted, there is a big difference between basic survival, and having material things such as a new ski boat. This was only an example to prove my point, that any person can successfully have or achieve *anything* they want simply by setting and following priorities. The ones highest on the list will be accomplished first, and so on down the line. Becoming physically fit and having the look you want will depend a lot on where you put it on your priority list. The further down, the further delayed the results become.

No one gets something for nothing. Good health is no exception. Just as in life itself, anything of value comes with sacrifice, work, and commitment. Sorry, no free-bee's.

****************** Hang In there! ******************

Are you still with me? Great! Now, I want to further educate you on a few more of those exercise essentials that are likely to influence the outcome of both your short and long term goals in regard to this fitness program. All are significant mental footnotes that will require you to think, and *Use Your Head*.

****

LET YOUR CONSCIENCE BE YOUR GUIDE

I think everyone has an inner directional guidance system telling them what and when to do something, sort of like a personal advisor. I like to call it "my little voice", more commonly referred to as your *conscience.*

Your conscience can be a powerful tool, which, if used in a positive manner, will almost always steer you in the right direction. Your conscience sends you many various decision-making choices everyday, only it is your choice whether or not to listen.

For example, your conscience helps to distinguish right from wrong, good from bad, as well as help measure self-worth. With regard to exercise, your conscience can also be very accurate at letting you know such things as whether or not you are slacking, cheating, or just being lazy during your workout period. It will let you know, deep down, how and when to better recognize such common, self-defeating habits that all too often steer you opposite of what you really know is best. "I'm just not in it, I'll do it tomorrow," or "That's good enough, I think I'll skip the last couple of exercises and quit early." Sound familiar?

But on the flip side, it will also send other important signals like "I don't feel very well, I honestly don't think I should exercise today" or "Whoa, I think I just pulled a muscle, maybe I'd better lay off of this muscle group for a little while until it feels better."

If you think about it, your conscience is also probably the best diet guide you have, but here again you have to honestly listen to it, then follow up.

So use this built-in tool you and I have. It's free, and if used right, can be an important addition to your "Physical Results" arsenal.

SORENESS

In beginning an exercise program, or perhaps switching to a different one, it's very likely you will probably experience a certain degree of soreness soon afterwards. The soreness I'm referring to here is *muscle* soreness. This occurs when muscle fibers are slightly strained or torn, which is quite normal when undertaking most any kind of new physical activity or exercise.

Here, a sore muscle resulting from exercise should be thought of as positive stimulation. It is your body's way of responding, reminding you your efforts have not been in vain. Welcome the feeling, bringing with it a sense of accomplishment and a new awareness of muscles long forgotten.

Do not be frightened, intimidated, or work too hard to avoid it. Instead, learn to read muscle soreness, be at one with it, and teach yourself how to use it to enhance the quality of your workouts.

For those inexperienced, there quite possibly will be a few times in the beginning when you feel so sore, that you honestly feel you should postpone or skip working out entirely, at least until the soreness goes away. But in truth, this is not always the case.

For example, take the day after your first workout. You could very well feel slight to moderately sore, probably intensifying later that afternoon. This is your rest day in accordance with the beginners program so you won't be doing any exercising anyway.

Usually, it is on the third day after that first workout before the soreness has reached its peak. At that point, you must take heart and hang in there. You still can complete your workout as scheduled (providing you have no **serious** pain or injury), even though your body seems to be telling your brain that it just can't make it while feeling so sore. But in all sincerity and in most cases, you can.

You will be pleasantly surprised to find that once you begin to **properly warm up** and have made it through that first set or first group of exercises, those stiff and sore sensations become easier to handle than when you first began only minutes before. Yes, it is still there, but at this point, it somehow becomes much easier to work through.

Therefore, it is recommended you proceed at a *moderate* level of intensity for this and the next workout later on. In other words, continue to exercise, but take it easy. Try not to push yourself too hard during these early stages. This will enable you to work through the first week safely, without skipping workouts or pulling muscles.

By the third or fourth day, your body will soon become accustom to the current work load, and the stiff and sore feeling should eventually begin to subside.

If you maintain a dedicated, **consistent** workout schedule, eventually you will experience little or no muscle soreness from then on. However, if you miss 5-7 days in a row, you may re-experience a certain degree of soreness all over again.

PAIN

Ouch! No one likes pain. But the sensation of pain is your body's most valuable feeling in determining a possible oncoming injury (not to be interpreted the same as soreness). Pain should never be ignored, but rather evaluated.

Instead, find out what is causing it and learn what it means. Your body is sending you signals for a reason. These signals are precautionary messages telling you to either slow down, continue, take a break, warm up some more, or stop, your ankle is really broken. The degree of pain you experience will aid you in determining how bad it really is.

The better you are able to evaluate pain and its relation to your body, the better understanding and control you will have in not only dealing with it, but avoiding it.

SET GOALS

One of the keys to any successful venture, again, whether it be health, sports, or finance, is the practice of setting goals. They are most generally fixed on paper or fixed in the mind.

In following our quest of physical fitness, the goals most commonly put on <u>paper</u> are usually those of desired pounds and inches. Record these personal goals, then pin up or place them where you will see them several times a day. The refrigerator, bulletin board, the bathroom mirror, I think you get the picture. Photographs also work well as motivational factors. Such concrete reminders will further help to keep your thoughts continually focused on the commitment you have made for yourself.

However, the goals you set in your <u>mind</u> should be in the form of self-visualization. **See** yourself positive. **See** yourself productive. **See** yourself happy.

For example, is there a certain look you want, a look that would not be afraid to wear a bathing suit? What about improving your athletic potential, breaking that school record, lowering your golf score, or being able to jog for 30 minutes without stopping? Perhaps reaching for a higher energy level would be nice, a way to bounce you over the rigors of day to day routines? What about improving your confidence and self-image, regaining that feeling-good-about-yourself attitude?

These questions and many others are great reasons to begin practicing self-visualization tactics. Tactics that train your subconscious into accepting whatever you hold in your mind and make it into reality. Because if your mind accepts your goals as being real, so will your body. Remember, "seeing is believing".

But whatever it is, make sure you define it. When a particular goal has been defined, only then is it much easier to control and evaluate progress. Whether it's reducing to a certain dress size or being able to knock in a home run on a weekend softball game, *setting goals brings **desire** just one step from **reality***. Believe in them, work toward them, and they **will** happen!

PATIENCE

Patience is something all of us fall short of from time to time. We all want results and we want them NOW. Unfortunately, a lack of patience seems to be just a part human nature.

It must be understood that improved fitness does not happen overnight. Nor does anything else of value worth having. With exercise, demanding new things from your body too quickly will most often cause it to rebel, possibly creating down time due to injury. (There's that "ouch" again!)

Having patience directly corresponds with your set goals, or in other words, learning to patiently achieve step B before jumping to step C. In essence, experiencing patience is very much like climbing a ladder, learning to take one step at a time, to reach the top.

.

WORKOUT PARTNER?

Having a workout partner is more a question of personal preference rather than a requirement. While some choose the solitary route, many others feel naked without one.

A good training partner should be someone with common goals and interests. It should be someone you can always depend on to be there, never one to fink out on a workout. Good workout partners help push and fire each other up. It is a person who will contribute positively and provide inspiration, while bringing a feeling of camaraderie and friendship. They can also be a big help in spotting you when lifting heavy or out jogging the "buddy system" way, in turn, ensuring a much safer environment.

If you already have a workout partner, play it safe and try to avoid over-competing with one another when lifting, running, whatever. Competition between friends is good only to a point, that is, until you begin to over-compete, thus sacrificing concentration and technique in an effort to match or beat your partners challenge. Instead, compete or *challenge,* if you will, each other to smooth, perfect repetitions and good form.

If you are married, including your spouse as a workout partner can be beneficial in many ways also. Exercising together not only keeps you both healthy and looking good, but allows that extra time together that is becoming harder and harder to find.

On the other hand, you may simply prefer to workout alone. I choose this to be my favorite way by virtue of many reasons. The first is the complete feeling of self-sufficiency. I depend on no one but myself for motivation and achievement of my desired goals. I will take credit for my own success, as well as my own failures.

Secondly, it allows me to spend less time between sets and with fewer distractions. This greatly improves concentration and helps maintain my sense of direction and focus.

In certain gym atmospheres, I also find going at it alone makes it much easier to jump in and complete a set on a machine or bench apparatus that is currently being used, without too much interruption to those with whom you are sharing. It simply allows you more flexibility in the continuation and scheduling of your training periods.

All in all, the question of whether or not to choose a workout partner becomes more a matter of personal preference, and that of meeting your individual needs.

FOOL ME ONCE - SHAME ON ME!

Sad but true, there is a common misconception still with us in our exercise world today on the topic of *spot reducing.* It's when one continually exercises or isolates one particular problem area, in a futile attempt to get rid of the unwanted fat deposits in that area.

How many times have you seen a man with a spare tire around his middle, cranking out a jillion sit-ups in an attempt to trim his protruding waistline, or a woman doing mega sets of leg lifts in an effort to rid the fatty deposits on her thighs and buttocks?

Be aware that fat does not belong to any one particular muscle group, rather, fat is in a group all its own.

By attempting to isolate one particular area, you only succeed in working the muscle **under** the fat, not the fat itself. Sorry, but contrary to what many still believe or so desperately want to believe, fat removal by selective spot reducing <u>does not work.</u>

Instead, fat is burned in the body, *randomly.* It will burn that which is most readily available at the time it is needed, however, not necessarily in the area you want. Unfortunately, and to the dismay of many, the waistline in men and the thigh-buttocks area in women are the last to go. This is primarily due to the natural genetic makeup in both sexes.

But genetics aside, it is the strength training/aerobic endurance exercises in combination with proper diet practices that provide the most fat burning benefits, NOT spot isolation exercises. It is important that you understand and accept this concept now, before mounting frustration sets in and you give up trying completely.

Hopefully, by gaining a healthier, overall understanding of how your body works, you will find it distinctively easier in reaching your physical goals.

GIMMICKS - SHAME ON YOU!

Spot reducing is one thing that, at least, shows an effort behind the motive. But falling prey to a gimmick is quite another story.

It's very disappointing to see so many lazy, desperate, gullible people, always searching for the easiest way possible to get into shape. People will buy and try just about anything, leaving our fitness world fraudulent and gimmick-ridden. People need to wake up and quit making millionaires out of these gimmick-inventing entrepreneurs and their marketing agents. For they, and they alone, will be the only ones to benefit from your despair, not you.

If in doubt, ask yourself why there are so many people out of shape in this country. If getting in shape was as easy as many of the advertising gimmicks promise, then almost everyone would be a vision of perfect health. Surely, you are not one to believe everything you see, hear or read. You know it's not possible to enter the fitness theater directly to center stage via the back door, without first paying the full price of admission out front. It's just not that easy.

Next time, all the time, always approach the aisle to fitness carefully, and **use your head**. Make sure you thoroughly research any health or fitness related gimmick, diet, or advertisement. There are so many out there, I will not even attempt to list them all.

Simply avoid those products promising fast, overnight results, and ones requiring little or no effort. Not only will they most likely end in failure and frustration, but could very well be unhealthy as well. Again, always use your head and good ol' common sense. Don't be another sucker. *If it sounds to good to be true, it probably is.*

GETTING INTO THE HABIT

Exercise

Habits are formed by repetition, and proper exercise is one that must be engaged in 3 days a week at the very least. Regular exercise should become second nature, so much so, that if you miss or skip your day for exercise, you experience a gnawing feeling of guilt and incomplacency.

Also, habitual exercise should not be limited to just one way of thinking either. For instance, making aerobics your only center of activity is now regarded as insufficient exercise for the 65% or so remaining muscles of the upper body.

Studies have shown that over the last several years those who have made aerobic exercise their only concern, have increased in cardiovascular endurance, BUT greatly lack in upper body strength needed for normal day to day activities. Not only is one limited to how much one should normally be able to lift, but as age increases, the bones of the body also become weak and brittle frequently causing shattered hips, ankles, and so forth.

That is why the incorporation of weight-bearing, **upper-body**, **strength training exercises** are so important (chapter nine). This type of training helps both firm and maintain muscle mass as well as increase bone strength and density, which can assist in the slow down, or possibly even reverse process of osteoporosis.

On the other side of the coin, and for those who basically live in the weight room, you should also know and understand, that weight training alone does not carry all of the essential benefits in one package either. Although most are aware of this common fact of fitness, there are many who still would rather confine themselves to just pushing weights, than having to sit on a stationary bike or join an aerobics class. But wanting and having that level of complete and total fitness purely dictates that everyone, bar none, involve themselves in some type **of aerobic activity** on a regular basis (chapter twelve).

Granted, there is and probably always will be, a distinct group separation between those who partake in aerobic exercises only, to those who choose solely to train with weights. Generally, you tend to have the aerobic fanatics in one corner and the weight-heads in the other. But both groups should ultimately accept that **good habits of exercise** go a little beyond any set group or standard, instead, <u>together</u> (aerobic exercise and weight training), they should all be incorporated and perceived as one.

Diet

As outlined in the previous chapter "Let's Eat", your results from even the best exercise program will be fewer and less dramatic if not complimented by good eating habits. I will not elaborate further regarding diet, for you should know by now of its importance.

Rest and Relaxation

Never get into the habit of continuously over-working yourself day in and day out. Your diet-exercise program will benefit most when accompanied by proper rest and recovery habits.

Believe it or not, this all-important recovery period after exercise is where most of the beneficial events from your earlier efforts actually take place, not during exercise. It's when the physiological after-effects kick in and work to expel wastes and toxins throughout the body, thus allowing it to again, repair, rebuild, and grow stronger.

Most experts say we need 7-9 hours of sleep, possibly more depending upon the amount of training involved. The absence of good rest is like a generator is to a battery. Without the ability to recharge, it will only be able to keep going so long before eventually becoming drained.

But physical recuperation is not the only consideration in an exercise program. Usually, after a few months of solid dedication and consistency in working out, it is also quite common to experience a certain degree of mental burnout. Most call it boredom. Although your body is physically able to carry on, many times your mind becomes exhausted and needs a rest too.

It is here, after about a four to six month period of faithful exercise, I recommend remedying the situation by *rewarding* yourself with a self-prescribed one to two week break or vacation, if you will. This consists of leaving your workout routine with no obligation at all regarding exercise. Some call it goofing off. I refer to it as "earned" time. Use this short, self-prescribed, time-out to kick back a little and recharge. It can make a big difference.

Or, if you feel uncomfortable about stopping all activity, try breaking up the monotony of regular exercise by getting involved in some other type of sporting activity, conventional or otherwise. It doesn't have to be overly hard or easy, just different. It's your opportunity to play and have some fun of a different kind.

Either way, this short break cleanses the mind and greatly restores that inner drive you had when first starting. In addition, it provides you with something to look forward to after a few months or so of hard work, sort of like being able to see the light at the end of the tunnel.

Just the fact that you know there is an end to it once in a while is a big motivator in itself. It is something we ALL need at one time or another. (You won't fall that far out of shape in that short a period of time, but it is probable that you will re-experience a slight to moderate stage of soreness and fatigue as you did in the beginning, but to a lesser degree.)

Although you have allowed yourself two weeks to goof off, some find it hard to wait that long. Many find themselves so refreshed and fired up after only a week, they find themselves back in their workout pattern again, more enthused than ever. Try it!

Positive Attitude

In order for you to maintain your life long commitment of health and fitness, it is critical that you somehow form a positive mental attitude towards exercise. Make it into a habit that can be carried with you at all times. Although difficult at times, the development and maintaining of this type of attitude will not only be instrumental in shaping your physical goals, but it will also do a lot to re-awaken many of your true, inner qualities and personality strengths that often become buried over time.

Besides, a physically fit person with an openly positive attitude regularly shows to be more in control of his or her surroundings. This foremost group of individuals *indirectly* send out messages of confidence and stability to those around them, such as an employer, co-worker, or a prospective client. They just seem to carry themselves a little differently than most, usually standing out in a crowd. In short, *a positive attitude will lead to positive returns.*

So say good-bye to the Bah-humbugs, instead, say hello to more Boy-howdies!

Independence

Independent habits lead to independent lifestyles. This doesn't imply isolation, but rather, habitual self-sufficiency. In exercise you must be somewhat independent in order to succeed. And much of how you succeed will be determined by how you measure your own independence.

I found this quote by Dr. Michael J. Asken in his book "Dying To Win", a good example of what the expression of independence means to me. Just what does it mean to you?

"Perhaps the thing I value most in life is my independence and my ability to be in control of my life. If you value your independence and truly want to control your own life, then you often have to make hard decisions. Being independent doesn't mean doing the opposite of what others advise you to do. Being contrary just means you are controlled in a different way. True independence, to me, means keeping control. Independent thinkers don't wear that independence on their sleeves or advertise it by their hair styles. They show it through their actions, which are often very quiet and unnoticed except by those around them who care to observe."

JUST BE YOURSELF!

Peer Pressure

Perhaps, one of the greatest enemies to any fitness program, is the element of peer pressure. Anywhere there is exercise, it seems to be present. In our schools, gyms, fitness facilities, even in our homes, there is a continued fear of how others will pass sentence.

It is here that I think most of us at one time or another, usually the guys, have stacked on more weight than we can possibly handle correctly. Usually, it's where proper weight training technique and direction get completely thrown out the window. Granted, some of it is purely due to competitiveness, but a considerable part of it is because of *peer pressure.* "Who's watching? Are they impressed? I've got to keep up, or, I know I can do more than he can", and so on. It's an invisible form of exercise paranoia that wreaks havoc on both mind and body, leading many to self-doubt and insecurity.

RESIST! Just be yourself, it's that simple. You're overall success will depend on it. It shouldn't matter whether you feel you are being compared, critiqued, or are simply made fun of, **you must avoid allowing any outside pressures to dictate the quality and outcome of your workouts**. This applies to those aerobic-oriented individuals as well. Always keep in mind your primary reason for exercising in the first place. It's for YOU, remember?

An Ego With A Heavy Appetite

Aside from peer pressure, strength testing, or legitimate power lifting competition, inside almost any weight training program, there is a familiar mind-set that still seems to prevail. One that suggests, **the heavier you lift, the greater the results**. It never fails! Sadly, this often misunderstood concept of lifting heavier, whether true or not, is usually determined more by ego manipulation, rather than true justification. It is here where we must start from scratch and re-define the concept of *heavy* lifting.

In essence, it's when one continues to use a resistance greater than what he or she can *properly* execute. But mention this to an accomplished ego-ciser and you may get a response like "I have to lift heavy, it makes me feel like I'm doing something," or "lifting heavy helps my confidence." To those people I ask, "define <u>heavy</u> for me."

Usually, they throw out some specific number, like 350 pounds for example. Or they express the need to lift 95 to 100 per cent of their max, and so on. Fine then, I have no quarrel with that, *as long as it can be done in at least 6 or more* <u>PERFECT</u> repetitions, <u>**WITHOUT BREAKING FORM**</u>.

That's right, you guessed it, they can't do it. Their EGO continues to tell them to stack it on, regardless of what they get out of it. To illustrate, take the squat or bench press exercise as an example. Many times you will notice an individual strut proudly while stacking on the plates. But also notice with each following set, his technique worsens every time more weight is added. So what's the point?

Don't get me wrong, *progressive resistance training* is where it's at when it comes to developing size and strength. For a muscle to grow, it must be exercised and put under a greater load than what it is normally used to lifting. But so much of the time and for whatever reason, one often deviates from the old, time-proven concepts of basic weight training technique, rather focusing in on mind games and other non-productive practices.

Next time you happen to be in a gym atmosphere, take a little extra time to observe those lifting around you. *Use your head* and learn to distinguish between what and what not to do. Under the circumstances, learn to control your ego, instead of allowing it to control you.

Role Models

In a somewhat similar situation, how many times have you noticed one who always enjoys strutting his stuff, usually those of the male gender? Perhaps an overly cocky attitude, even to the point of obnoxious? Again, usually lifting heavier than what he is normally capable of doing right in hopes of gaining attention from all those around? You've seen them. This kind of annoying behavior happens all the time in schools and gyms all over the country.

Confidence is one thing, and it is unfortunate that these types of individuals cheat themselves so. But even more unfortunate, are the ones working out next to them who have a tendency to follow their example by using them as *role models*.

Following one's lead or patterning yourself in this manner will not only cause you to lose efficiency in training, but also lose a few friends in the process. So, before you get too carried away with putting someone up on a pedestal, always analyze the situation then ask yourself, does this person physically look like he knows what he is doing or talking about? Does he follow his own advice? He may have big arms and chest, but judging from his stomach area, it's doubtful that he seriously works his abdominals or even knows the meaning of a proper diet.

Simply put, stay away from the "wannabe's". Allow them to continue fooling themselves. Instead, seek out and follow the advice from someone who IS successful and obviously looks the part they represent. You will find these kind of people to be more than happy in sharing their knowledge and experience with you. Follow their *exact* path, and you too will be successful. Here, you cannot fail!

WOMEN ON WEIGHTS

Hey gals! On your marks, get set, whoa? Unfortunately, there still remains a majority of you out there who hold the notion that lifting weights will make you bulky and unfeminine. Still, others become scared off by other related misconceptions or just plain, bad advice. Sure, there are those select few who seem to have more natural ability to develop than most others, but one must not immediately group themselves into this unique category without first doing a little research on their own.

Typically, what comes to the mind of many is the professional female body builder, carrying with it visions of muscled perfection. This elite class of athlete develops and maintains their body to a much higher degree than what most refer to as normal standards. Extreme dieting, intense determination, and hours upon hours of training is looked upon as nothing short of routine in their rigors of day to day life.

But, it must be emphasized, these and the ones you see in muscle magazines for instance, whatever you may think of them, are obviously on a professional level. Ninety-nine percent of all others never get that far, nor even want to. If this is you, worry not. Now know that it IS possible to lift weights and not bulk out.

First off, women must realize that their own body make up will not allow them to generate much size, no matter how hard they may try. The hormones for building any kind of noticeable mass are there, but not in the quantities needed. Unlike the male for example, whose levels of testosterone (the hormone most responsible for muscle development) far exceed that of any female. For this reason alone, one should not have to worry. If, by any chance you have any doubts, stay with higher repetitions using light to moderate weight, while maintaining perfect exercise form and of course, watch your diet.

Fortunately, for women today, there are more and more discovering the benefits and advantages that come with incorporating weight training exercises to their workout schedule. Most are surprised to find just how much better they look and feel after giving it a try.

Keep in mind, the muscles of the body is what gives it it's shape and figure, and for most women that is their primary concern. Muscles provide not only strength for movement, but also create those eye-pleasing curves along with basic normal body context.

So, the old stereotype of men only in the weight room is gone, giving way to a whole new and refreshing atmosphere. Those who have taken advantage of such opportunities will tell you, *you've been missing out.*

FEELING OUT OF IT?

More times than not, exercising will be the last thing you'll want to do. Although this is no secret to anyone, it does eventually happen, so don't feel too much like the Lone Ranger when it happens. Tonto will tell you, "You with plenty good company".

Without doubt, diminishing intensity levels along with the monotony of exercise can make it hard for anyone to pep themselves up before each and every workout. This is where your conscience enters as a valuable tool. It will, most assuredly, step in at the proper time and let you know whether you truly feel ill, injured, or accept other reasons that are legitimate for skipping.

But by and large, whatever the reason for wanting to "blow it off", it's usually nothing more than a lethargic mood swing or Ho-hum attitude that brings with it erratic, and inconsistent workouts. Myself included. I am no different and regularly find myself NOT in the mood or state of mind to begin my scheduled workout session either.

Nevertheless, it is a critical hump we all must learn to get over, not just once or twice, but time and time again. It won't be easy, and waiting around for it to go away rarely ever happens. So, regardless of what your mood is at the time, you've got to force both mind and body to:

JUST... START... ANYWAY...

Just do it, trust me! Just start! It's the ONLY way! You will be pleasantly surprised to find out that somewhere after warming up and finishing the first set or two of the first exercise, you gain back that determined, fired up feeling that you seemed to lack only minutes before. Oddly, it somehow works itself out.

Consequently, every time you succeed in conquering those pesky, negative signals that are quick to kill any fitness program, you mentally grow stronger and more in control of your exercise habit as a result.

Over time, you should try to get to the place your workouts become less and less of a conscious effort, eventually reverting into an *automatic mode*. Again, just doing it! In so doing, you will find the burden of exercise much easier to handle time after time.

MISCELLANEOUS THOUGHTS

- Wherever you find a muscle it is there for a reason, and thus a need for movement. Use it, or you loose it!

- The many benefits you receive from exercise are not permanent, once you stop, so do the benefits. That is why it becomes increasingly important to make it a life long commitment.

- The act of exercise often creates a steam-rolling effect. As body aesthetics develop, so too, does one's self-esteem. This, then, gives birth to a self-induced feeding frenzy. One that continues to cycle as long as both (mind & body) remain nourished.

- *Use your head*, listen to it and your conscience. If you do, it won't let you down.

- On a final note;

  Every so often, you may notice one that naturally sticks out in a crowd, one that immediately sends out signals of vibrant health and an enviable physique, one who is full of energy and positive in their attitude. They are the small percentage of individuals in our society that look, act, and are successful, taking full control of their lives both in and out of the gym. This exclusive group stands out and above the rest by taking extra good care of their health and well-being, in turn, leaving nothing more to prove, except only to be themselves. Now quiz yourself, *how do you think you come across to others?*

CHAPTER SIX:

TRADE TOOLS AND TECHNIQUE

As you probably know by now, the required tools of the trade come in a wide variety of shapes, sizes, and price ranges. This, along with the process of determining what equipment is required, in addition to what one needs to know, can be quite a large hurdle to overcome. For that purpose, I have put together a list of only those items and related concepts in which I feel are most fundamental to your success.

(If, however, you consider yourself to be somewhat experienced in exercise basics, feel free to skim over that which you are already familiar and move on. *Make sure you stop and put on the brakes when you get to the sub-chapter "Exercise Technique",* because from here on out is where the heart and lifeblood of this program really begins.)

EXERCISE EQUIPMENT

Good news! The exercise program in this book can be done at home or in a semi, to fully-equipped gym. You should make your choice by not only what equipment is available, but one in which you will feel most comfortable. Consideration should also be made in the location or facility you have chosen, to be the best suited at fitting into your lifestyle, yet, with the assurance that all personal goals will be met.

Health Clubs: yes, no, maybe?
Most any reputable gym or health club organization should have everything you need as far as facilities and apparatus are concerned in order for you to adequately follow this particular exercise program. Additional considerations, such as child-care services, personal evaluations, club hours, and properly certified and available staff members should also be a part of your inquiries.

If a health spa or gym is unavailable, or just not for you, you may want to think about exercising at home. Personally, I have had by far, many more gung-ho, up-beat, and productive workouts at home, than in any gym or club I have ever belonged to. So never feel pressured into joining a fitness facility just because you believe it is the only way to attain quality workouts.

Plus the fact, if you consider the cost of some of the club membership prices, it may be economically feasible and rather more to your liking to invest in your own equipment and exercise at home.

Hardware

For the weight training segment of this program, you will need a barbell/dumbbell assortment, preferably at least a 110 pound set. Prices range from relatively cheap to somewhat expensive and can be purchased at most sporting goods stores. (Chapter thirteen covers the weight *machine-oriented* program).

An example of a less expensive set would be the plastic, plaster-filled kind (under $25). A little more elaborate, but better quality, is the iron plate "Olympic" set ($175-$300+). Both do the same job with personal preference being the deciding factor. While your at it, make it a point to purchase a curling bar and four extra 2 1/2 pound plates to allow you further weight variance during certain dumbbell exercises. They are not always included in the basic package, but there is a good chance you will need them at one time or another.

The same goes in choosing a weight bench. The prices range from very cheap to very expensive. Choose a bench that is at least in the moderate price range. The cheaper models are usually inferior in quality and overall structural stability.

Furthermore, I recommend you choose a bench equipped with an adjustable back support, one that can lie flat or can be propped up to any one of a variety of angled positions. Add to that, an attached combination leg extension/leg curl apparatus. That should do it.

There are many other fancy extras and add-ons that are available, but generally unnecessary at this point. If you look around, you can find a good all-purpose bench for around $200. It is important that you have access to this kind of semi-purpose bench either in your home or your favorite gym, in order to properly execute this particular program as well as most other exercise programs respectively. It may seem like quite an investment, but in comparison to what most people spend their money on, this investment in health will continue to pay dividends throughout a lifetime.

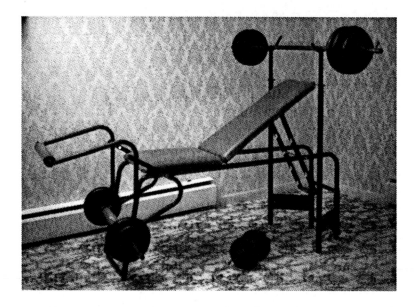

(Those individuals who are more concerned with losing fat weight <u>initially</u>, should lean more toward the tools and concepts defined in chapter twelve.)

Other Tools

There are many other exercise extra's out there that may or may not be useful in aiding you in your quest for a better body. Tools such as mirrors, straps, belts, gloves and other related exercise equipment. Although it never hurts to be open to new things, you will find most of the fancy extras generally unnecessary and considered non-essential items. However, it is up to you to weigh the plusses and minuses accordingly, making it purely an option on your part.

Using such common-place items as a mirror could be one example of a useful tool, **IF** used for the right purpose. Mirrors are very helpful in analyzing one's technique during exercise, among targeting troubled areas. However, I strongly recommend that you avoid getting into the habit of *constantly* using a mirror with the exception of only once in a while. I find it greatly decreases your level of concentration over the long run, stealing your thoughts and concentration from where the emphasis should be, *inside* each particular muscle you are working. This happens most often in gym atmospheres where entire walls have been mirrored, a dedication to both the narcissistic, as well as the genuine troubleshooters.

Wrist straps are another consideration in exercise tool and gym attire. Made from 1" - 2" inch wide strips of heavy cloth nylon, some lifters use them as an anchor or crutch to aid in gripping a variety of weight bars and other apparatus during various pulling exercises. Securely wrapped around the lower part of a lifters wrist on down around the bar itself, these wrist straps allow one to lift heavier amounts of weight than one would normally be able to do properly. Others prefer to use them simply because of the enhanced isolation they receive when targeting a particular muscle group.

Unfortunately, many of those who make a habit of using them should also be aware, that by relying on just such a tool or crutch, also tends to rob the forearm and hand muscles of proper strength distribution and development. It is imperative to always try and maintain a determined effort toward ample proportion and balance of body conditioning. Unless you plan to include additional wrist and forearm exercises, I generally find the use of wrist straps unnecessary and less rewarding in the long run.

Another tool of the trade is the use of lifting belts. There are those who automatically associate weight training with the need to purchase one, either due to legitimate reasons, such as increased back support and stability, or simply because everyone else has one. These belts are usually made of heavy leather or high-tech synthetic nylon, and are durable, extra wide, and a common piece of exercise apparel among most all free weight gyms. They are widely considered an essential tool towards safer lifting.

Nevertheless, lifting belts should not be perceived to be this "must have, can't do without it" item. In most cases, throughout it's continual use, it basically provides the user with a false sense of security, and if one is lucky, possibly only a little extra in back support, no more. Often, those who wear them throughout each and every workout, whether they need it or not, eventually lead themselves into a feeling of utter dependency upon their use.

In truth, substituting these belts for support tends to indirectly take away from the coordinated effort and muscle stimulation normally provided by the abdominal and lower back muscles. It even becomes possible for the muscles of the back and stomach area to *weaken* from lack of use, in turn, reverting back to square one.

To some extent, there is a legitimate side to wearing one. The use of these belts is most often accepted when lifting exceptionally heavy weight or during competitive power lifting competitions. Those who fit into these categories are lifting large amounts of weight where there happens to be a considerable amount of inner and outer physical stress, with a higher than average chance of serious injury. (Such things are not part of this program.)

In summary, if you are one with certain physical problems or perhaps just a beginner, use whatever tool you need to acquire the balance and strength necessary to properly execute weight lifting exercises *safely*. But, if you are an athlete in training or athletically inclined, in the long run, avoid getting hooked on the need for such additional support. Rather, train freely without any crutches or exer-aids. Repetitive training in this free-form fashion greatly increases your sense of inner balance, in addition to the overall enhancement of strength and body coordination. Be free!

WHAT TO WEAR?

Exercise Apparel
There may be a question as what to wear during your workout. In most cases, you want to wear something loose and comfortable, something non-restricting (nothing so tight that it decreases blood flow), with freedom of movement at all times. This becomes even more important in the older age groups.

Beyond this, it's completely up to you as long as you keep fashion in the workout place reasonable. At times, fashionable sports-wear becomes unpractical and/or uncomfortable, although still self-important to many. Often, I find that the person who is worried more about how they look in their fashionable exercise-wear than in working out, are there for the wrong reason anyway. You must decide where to draw the line on what you wear in order to meet your own needs and comfort. Above all, be comfortable when working out.

Weather Permitting
Deciding on what to wear during exercise depends a lot on climatic weather conditions and the type of exercise undertaken. Much of which is determined by common sense. But the basic guidelines to follow for proper exer-wear, is to wear clothes that will absorb sweat and have the ability to dissipate heat. Cotton usually works the best for indoor activity, and is among the most comfortable. Stay away from such artificial fibers such as Polyester. This material has a tendency not to absorb as well as some of the synthetic fiber outfits.

For outdoor activity, such synthetic products seem to do a good job in transporting moisture away from your skin, rather than just absorbing and staying wet against your skin. Waterproof clothing is another option available for outdoor consideration. Again, necessity will determine your needs.

Shoes

Choosing a good pair of shoes is just as important as clothing selection. You should choose a shoe that best fits the sport or activity you undertake. And regardless of the activity, I recommend you not skimp too cheaply in this area. Cheaply made shoes commonly lead anywhere from mild discomfort, to severe inflammation of the lower joints and back. Inferior footwear has shown to be the common denominator to many fitness-related injuries. Believe it! It's well worth a few extra bucks to further insure yourself against possible injury and still have something with lasting quality.

If you feel a need for more individualized counseling on what to wear, seek out a reputable sporting goods advisory expert.

WHEN TO EXERCISE

Adjust To Your Meals

Just about any time of the day is a good time to exercise, except right before or soon after you have just eaten. Working out during this particular time frame tends to make you feel sluggish and lazy, a "just not in it attitude". But more importantly, it adds a considerable amount of stress on the heart.

For after you have just eaten, the heart is working harder than normal in order to send additional blood to the digestive tract to aid in the breakup and utilization of food during the body's normal digestion process. If you were to start exercising during this time, the heart would not only have to work harder to supply the digestive tract, but also work to supply that extra needed energy and oxygen for your muscles, in turn, creating an unnatural overload of your bodily functions.

Instead, give your body at least 1 1/2 hours of digestion time, *before* exercising. The same goes with right after exercise. Here again, give yourself somewhere around an hour or so afterwards to allow your body a chance to cool down. By taking such things as your eating timetable into consideration during the planning stages of your exercise schedule not only makes the exercise regime more comfortable, but much more safe and profitable to boot.

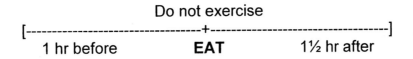

Do not exercise

[--------------------------------+--------------------------------]

1 hr before   **EAT**   1½ hr after

Set It Up

Setting up a workout schedule to your liking, yet still have the ability to fit it in and around your present lifestyle will take time, patience, and a bit of experimentation. Especially, in this not-enough-hours-in-a-day world in which we are all subjected. But having a set, specific schedule is a must!

One who tries to *find* time to exercise is never really successful, but the one who *plans* for it, IS.

For instance, *plan* a consistent time everyday that you can exercise, maintain a job, and still have time to spend with your family, friends, or any other of life's many projects and opportunities. Preferably, always at the same time at the same place. If you don't, if you continue to remain overly flexible with your schedule, you'll probably end up flexing your way right out of fitness.

When you finally create one that works, STICK WITH IT!

Recuperation: Anaerobic vs. Aerobic

When breaking down muscle through exercise, one must also recognize the need for rest and recovery, especially when it comes to weight training versus aerobic training. Although both require a certain recovery period, it is weight training that will require more of a patterned time-frame.

This is due to the constant break down of muscle tissue during the repetitive, weight-bearing motions of an-aerobic exercise. A rigorous, but natural process one must undergo to build strength and flexibility.

But, by pushing yourself too hard for too long, or working the same muscle or muscle group everyday without time for recuperation, without doubt, will eventually lead one down the slow path of deterioration, NOT increased productivity. So here again, more is not always better.

Therefore, the standard to go by will be no less than 48 hours between weight training workouts for the same muscle group. With few exceptions, a standard most weight programs still use today. A good example would be a Monday, Wednesday, Friday program, each providing at least a day rest in between.

EXERCISE TECHNIQUE

Speed Of Exercise

You should know and understand by now that there is a precise and correct way to train with weights. Know also that there is a precise and correct way of doing each movement. The speed in which you perform each repetition is an important part of that movement.

You should avoid fast, quick, jerky movements, replacing them instead with smooth, deliberate motions, maintaining constant control at all times.

Normally, speed of the upward lift of each exercise will take care of itself, providing you are using the correct amount of weight to begin with. Choosing how fast you can lift the weight is usually out of your hands, and most often that of "barely".

Aside from this, you do have more of a choice during the lowering phase. When lowering, YOU maintain control of the decent, disallowing the weights to pull or push YOU down. Force your muscles to uncoil slowly, thus maintaining a slight resistance over the entire repetition. Generally, lower at about half the speed in which you were able to lift.

Again, the key here will be upon control. Dropping the weight contributes little in the development of strength, and in some cases, increases your chance of injury to the muscles and tendons.   Eventually, and with a little time and effort on your side, your body will soon settle into its' own groove or rhythm, making the efforts of exercise safer and more profitable.

Breathing Habits

Yes, there is a right way and a wrong way to breathe when doing resistance-type exercises. I have found most of those I have instructed down through the years begin with bad exercise breathing habits. In fact, more times than not, you would find them doing just the opposite of how it should be done.

Technically, you should exhale on positive resistance and inhale on negative resistance. This means you should always exhale during the exertion or lifting phase of any exercise, while slowly and smoothly inhaling when lowering.

Perhaps in simpler terms, I like to instruct my students to think of it as "blowing the weights up." Visualize the barbells as big balloons. In order to get these balloons afloat and up in the air you must take a deep breath and physically blow them upward.

If done wrong, you present a greater amount of undue stress upon the cardiovascular system. The danger factor varies with each individual and their present physical condition, ranging from minor problems all the way up to a possible heart attack.

Nevertheless, proper breathing technique is much like exercise technique expressed earlier, it should be developed into a rhythm. Something you eventually don't even have to think about.

If all else fails and you are still in doubt, focus your emphasis on exhaling when lifting *anything,* whether it be a heavy sack of groceries or simply re-positioning the living room couch. Blow those weight up! The rest will come with practice.

Cheating

Cheating is a term used when one attempts to complete a repetition in the easiest way possible, by bypassing part, or most of the range of a particular muscle or muscle group. It is when one jerks, bounces, or swings the weights, using speed and momentum to initiate or complete each lift.

Cheating is very common for several reasons. One is not knowing that there is a right or wrong way in the first place.

Secondly, lack of concentration and proper technique during exercise has again, in many instances been **de**-emphasized, a habitual mind-set that seems only concerned with how many repetitions get done, rather than *how it gets done.*

And thirdly, there is again the reality of peer pressure. The pressure of being around others who are able to use heavier weight, thus providing one a feeling of having to add more weight than he or she can lift properly, whereby resorting to cheating.

All in all, when you cheat in anything, you end up cheating yourself. Exercise is no different. So, stay clean, stay honest, and stay productive!

Isolation

As I have stated earlier, your mental focus during each repetition of each exercise is critical. You must *isolate* yourself mentally, and become one with ONLY that particular muscle or muscle group you are working. All other non-involved body parts like the hand and facial muscles should be as relaxed as possible.

Think of nothing else. This is not the time to allow the mind to wander. Not a time to allow outside worries or problems to interfere with the intensity of your thought patterns. All attempts should be towards recruiting **every strand** of muscle fiber possible in and throughout the targeted body part.

Full Range Of Motion

As you proceed throughout each of the following weight training exercises, you will notice each one is specifically instructed to be executed through its fullest range of motion. A crucial training technique that ensures the stimulation of the entire muscle, thus promoting size, full-range strength, definition, and crucial joint flexibility. Add to this, the drastic reduction of the chance of becoming "muscle bound".

For it is this troublesome notion of becoming "muscle bound", that frequently comes to the mind of many when contemplating any kind of weight program. More often, it happens to the individual who constantly exercises a muscle or muscle group in a fixed position.

This in no way refers to being strapped or belted down to some fancy gym apparatus either. Actually, it comes as a result from executing poor form and technique during each exercise movement, a tendency of only going part or half way.

By continuously exercising in this manner, the connective tissue of the muscle begins to adapt to this fixed position, never being allowed to completely stretch. This eventually leads to a shortening of the muscle, which in turn limits the potential range of motion of that respective joint.

Only by exercising each muscle or muscle group through their fullest range of motion, in conjunction with various stretching exercises will you ensure yourself from becoming muscle bound. Remember, a longer, more flexible muscle will always be a much stronger, healthier muscle.

GYM JARGON

And finally, regardless of how, when, or where you exercise, one should be reasonably familiar with some of the basic terms and concepts associated with exercise. Here are but a few.

- A *Workout Program* is a set order of exercise or group of exercises **that one chooses in accordance to his or her own goals and intensity levels.**

- A *Repetition* (or rep) is the actual act or full movement of exercise, in any one given set. Usually done repeatedly for a required number of times.

- A *Set* is a specific or prescribed number of repetitions, executed throughout it's entirety. For our purposes, and in corresponding with the following weight training program provided in this book, a set will always be 6-12, 8-12, or 10-15 repetitions, except where otherwise specified.

- *Progressive Resistance Training* is when one continues to add a certain amount of weight with each following set.

- Never confuse weight <u>lifting</u> with weight <u>training</u>. *Weight lifting* is a sport, in which one attempts to lift a maximum amount of weight in the easiest manner possible, relying on speed and technique to bypass most of the range of the muscle. A good example would be a competitive Olympic power lifter performing a clean-and-jerk.

- *Weight training* on the other hand is just the opposite. It is the art of building the body, by isolating and working the muscles through their full range of motion, using just the right amount of resistance so that you can safely do each repetition technically perfect. Weight training will give you the maximum physical response for the effort put out, such as strength, shape, tone, and muscle size. The elite body builder and the main concept of this book are two good examples.

- A *spotter* is a partner or friend that watches over you when lifting heavy or in certain risky situations. If help is needed, the spotter is right there.

- Getting *pumped up* is a phrase used after having just worked a particular muscle or area of the body, as a result the lifter experiences a full, warm, even bigger feeling, due to the concentration of blood in that area.

- "Boy, I felt a good *burn* on that one." A burn in this case, usually occurs during a repetitive movement towards the end of a set, when it feels as though the muscle you are exercising is on fire.

- The *smooth* look refers to an individual that has little or no muscle definition.

- The more *defined* person is one that shows good muscularity.

- The individual described as looking *cut* or *cut up*, simply means that he or she is extremely well defined.

- The very ultimate is the *ripped* look. A rare body type that is so well cut and defined, it carries a resemblance of an anatomy chart.

Other terms and/or phrases used in the exercise world many times include body parts lingo, usually in the form of basic muscle terminology. Whether you are physically active or not, you no doubt have heard words like bicep, hamstring, pectorals, and so forth. This same style of jock talk is also frequently used in short, abbreviated slang form, each corresponding to a particular muscle or muscle group. (Abs, Pecs, Delts, etc.)

The ones frequently used most are shown in the following illustration, each designating where that particular muscle is located and the proper name of that muscle in parenthesis. Familiarizing yourself with this style of jargon is not all that crucial, but it never hurts.

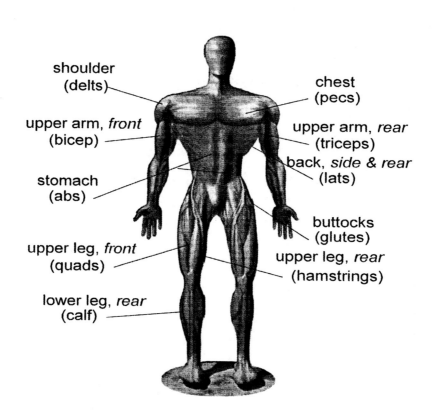

shoulder (delts)

chest (pecs)

upper arm, *front* (bicep)

upper arm, *rear* (triceps)

back, *side & rear* (lats)

stomach (abs)

buttocks (glutes)

upper leg, *front* (quads)

upper leg, *rear* (hamstrings)

lower leg, *rear* (calf)

CHAPTER SEVEN:

SUCCESS IS "M.E.T."

Why spend years trying to build and sculpt your body, when you could achieve the same thing in only a matter of months?

As promised, the art of maximizing your efforts to equal the time spent exercising is now closer to reality. Introducing:

MAXIMUM EFFICIENCY TRAINING

This newly developed concept known as *Maximum Efficiency Training* (or M.E.T.) is one of the highest priorities of this book. These remaining principals that follow have all been drawn from the time-tested basics of bodybuilding fundamentals and practical application.

These simple, but precise strategies assembled here in "M.E.T.", will clearly benefit anyone who faithfully puts forth the effort to improving their strength and shape. It is a continual, repeated attempt by the author, to eliminate any and all wasted time and effort of this particular weight training program, *in comparison to all others.*

What it all comes down to, is that it should be everyone's objective to get the utmost out of each and every exercise period, for the **AMOUNT OF TIME THEY PUT IN**. Going forward instead of backward. Being able to exit the workout with that reassured feeling of knowing your time and effort was maximized, used to the fullest. Being able to say to yourself, "Whew, that was another good one." Anything less should leave you feeling unfulfilled and bearing a guilty conscience. THAT is the basis for the concept of M.E.T.

So, before venturing any further into the following weight training program, it would be highly beneficial for one to review, instill, and emphasize in your mind, these following crucial components of "M.E.T." found here in this special chapter, in addition to those found throughout earlier parts of this book. They make all the difference.

M.E.T
Maximum Efficiency Training

a) *Use Your Head*   (chapter 5)
b) *Full Range Of Motion during each repetition*   (chapter 6)
c) *Isolation* of each movement   (chapter 6)

d) *Follow Instructions To The Letter*
e) use the *Flex* technique
f) proper *Set Intervals*
g) *Train To Failure*
h) use the *Troubleshooting* guide accordingly

FOLLOW INSTRUCTIONS TO THE LETTER

Have you ever bought something that was stamped "some assembly required?" Like most of us who have, it's easy, at first, to allow impatience and enthusiasm to take over, thus giving way to a brief glance or quick skim over the step-by-step instruction sheet. You know, jump right in and start slapping things together. Though you honestly thought you knew what you were doing, it usually turns out that you should have followed the instructions a little more closely. Here, the situation is no different.

If you are to get the promised results out of this particular exercise program, you must follow the methods of instruction *to the letter.* Remember, no shortcuts. Everything mentioned is vital to reaching your goals. Not one concept or thought process can be overlooked or taken lightly.

But be forewarned! In the beginning it is possible that much of what is mentioned in this particular rendition of, "some assembly required", may not come about as planned. To fully understand or feel all that you think you should right from the get-go, probably won't happen as fast as you would like.

But with a little patience, persistence, and practice, it will *grab you like nothing you've ever felt before.* When this begins to happen, those long-awaited results you've been looking for won't be far behind.

Successfully following a good workout program will be like following a recipe to bake a cake. If you neglect to follow precisely as instructed, neither the cake nor you, will turn out the way you want.

AGAIN, USE YOUR HEAD

Stop right here! I recommend you go back and re-read the first part of chapter five called, "USE YOUR HEAD". Then come back here and proceed. Instill in your mind the importance of mental concentration and willpower. Again, this alone, will be the most important concept to be learned from this book.

TAKE IT OFF!

How can I express the importance of this next concept with as much emphasis as is necessary, for you, the reader, to take seriously, other than to just say it?

........"TAKE IT OFF!"........

That's right, take it off! Reduce the amount of weight you normally use during each exercise and replace it with much lighter resistance to start.

I know, this goes entirely against the way you have been taught or have been doing it up to this point, but far too many are getting started on the wrong foot. Sadly, I place much of the blame on those who's job it was to teach us right the first time; specifically, coaches. Not all coaches, but quite a few.

From junior high on up, many of our fitness mentors are still missing the point of what true weight *training* is all about. The problem is that the perfection of exercise technique is being replaced with "the more weight, the better" attitude. *"That's it Tommy, come on, you can get it. Bounce that sucker up there. Good job! Now who's next?"* Get the picture?

This type of mentality, or should I say, lack of attention, leads to further cheating in technique such as bouncing, jerking, or swinging of the weights. Not only are results much harder to find and injury likely, but hard to break habits are formed in this early learning process making the long road ahead rough and bumpy.

In essence, weight resistance should be used only as a **tool** towards reaching our physical goals. Tools that are essential in order to build, sculpt, tone, and strengthen. Thus, *the amount of weight* used during each exercise should be perceived as much a tool, as a hammer and saw is to build a house. Just as a hammer isn't used to cut wood or a saw to drive a nail, the amount of weight should not be used for anything other than its obvious purpose. Simply stated, if not used correctly, the job will not get done correctly.

Therefore, for our purposes, the amount of weight at this time is *irrelevant* and will take care of itself later on. It shouldn't matter whether you are pushing 2000 pounds or only 2, so long as you **get that house built**, built like a rock.

If you are just a beginner, pick a weight that you think you will be able to do successfully. At that *point drop the weight even more,* to a point you believe the resistance to be too easy. This specific starting point will ensure you have chosen a correct starting weight. If not, you can always add. As the rule goes, it is better to start with too light a weight, than too heavy.

If you are somewhat experienced in weight training, I insist that you try following the method if you haven't already.

Decrease the weight you normally use for each exercise by as much as 1/3 to 1/2, and keep it there, **at the same weight for each successive set.** Do not add or subtract. Instead, place more emphasis on using your MENTAL MUSCLES throughout each and every movement. You will not only be amazed in the difference you will feel, but also the ease in which your mind is able to isolate each movement of every muscle.

Later, when you are able to *PERFECTLY* execute more than the required number of repetitions as outlined in this program, <u>only then should you add weight and proceed accordingly</u>.

Unless you are a competitive power lifter or engaged in strength testing, it becomes highly impractical for most of us to push unnecessary poundage while sacrificing proper form.

So, Take It Off! This process of finding just the right amount of weight for each exercise will happen only when you learn to interpret and listen more to what your body is telling you, again, rather than listening to your pride or ego.

KEEP IT THERE

Once you have made it through the experimentation process of trying to find the optimum amount of weight for each exercise, find it, and then *keep it there*! Do not add or subtract any more weight once you find yourself able to successfully complete the required number of repetitions for each set, regardless of how many sets you plan to do.

This is quite unlike other programs that dictate you add weight with each corresponding set, again, setting the stage for an increase in cheating and poor form.

Depending upon which program level you have chosen, your only concern should be that of selecting the proper weight resistance that will allow you to stay, at least, in the 6-12 repetition range throughout each and every set. (If this becomes a problem, see the subtitle "Beginner's Last Call" located at the very end of "Troubleshooting".)

I repeat, once the muscles begin to adapt and you find yourself eventually exceeding the 12 or 15 rep maximum, or in other words, finding that particular exercise to be *overly easy*, only then is it permissible to add more weight.

SET INTERVALS

A common mistake many make when weight training, is taking too much time between sets. Simply put, they get too much rest. Don't get me wrong, you do need rest, but only a certain amount, especially with regard to "set intervals".

There are traditionally two different objectives one has had to choose from when trying to determine how much one should rest between each set;

One, is by using light resistance with little or no rest, thus emphasizing more in the direction of definition and endurance training.

The other, is by using heavier resistance with more rest (or full recovery). The emphasis and direction here is towards greater strength.

Good news! This program allows one to cut it down the middle and get the benefit of both worlds, and yet, without going to the extremes of either one. Simply follow this specialized rest guide.

<u>Rest Between Sets</u>

Beginners: As long as needed
Intermediate: 1 1/2 - 2 minutes
Advanced: 1 minute

(Note the exceptions; 1) poor physical condition 2) some of the larger muscle groups may require more recovery time than some of the smaller groups. Here, Squats could be considered an example of a longer recovery exercise.)

Make sure you carry a wrist watch or are able to monitor the second hand of a clock on a nearby wall. Disciplining oneself in this manner can be at times, fairly intense. So be patient and use caution. But keep an eye on that second hand. The time to start each new set comes around faster than you might think, so be ready.

If confusion still persists, a good rule to go by is **as soon as you catch your breath,** you should be ready to go again, no longer.

By conditioning yourself to train in this way will not only help prevent long, drawn-out, inconsistent workouts, but further ensures you to gain maximum productivity in strength, muscle development, body toning, and definition, **without spending all day in the gym.**

FLEX METHOD

Bingo! That's what you'll say to yourself after incorporating the *flex method* into your exercise technique. You MUST remember to <u>flex</u> (squeeze or tighten) each corresponding muscle or muscle group you are working, at the top end of each exercise repetition (the point at which the most contraction occurs). Not once-in-a-while, not every other set, and not just when you feel like it, but **each ...and ...every ...repetition.** Actually challenge yourself to try and stimulate as many of the individual muscle fibers as possible that make up the targeted area.

Try this:
Place both hands directly in front of your chest with the palms flat against each other and fingers extended out and away from the body (the same position one might have during a prayer).

Next, try to press them together as if you were attempting to crush or flatten some object between them. Each time, make sure you hold that tension momentarily in order to feel the upper chest muscles tighten and contract. (Sometimes referred to as an isometric exercise.)

Feel it? That is what one should normally expect to feel during any one of a variety of upper chest exercises. To me, this is what going through the motions feels like. Granted, you are getting something done, but only a fraction of what is possible.

NOW, using the same hand position, *extend your arms completely* out in front of you. Again, attempt the same crushing effort as you did before only this time you should notice an amazing difference between the two techniques.

Notice the drastic impact those same chest muscles experience by not only changing technique a little, but also how much more the mind is able to tie in to the large and small muscles alike, thereby creating a sense of fullness and personal accomplishment that can only be achieved through targeted exercise motion. NOW THAT'S ISOLATION. THAT'S FLEXING. THAT'S SUCCESS!

TRAINING TO FAILURE

If you're not *training to failure*, you are failing to train.

That's right. For those who consider themselves high achievers, the concept of "training to failure" is another must do. Although this is nothing new or innovative, it is hopefully something you've been doing all along throughout your weight training ritual. Quite simply, continue to work each muscle or muscle group until it ceases to function normally, thereby reaching a state of total fatigue. In other words, until the targeted muscle can do no more, rep by rep, set by set.

And just as in anything of this nature, caution is the key. Especially for those starting out. It is suggested you work up to this concept gradually, allowing yourself time to learn about the body and how it will respond to various levels of training intensity.

However, if you are interested in nothing more than simple body maintenance and possess no practical need for such intensity, disregard this concept and proceed at a level that best fits you and your outlined goals.

LARGE TO SMALL

The ordered layout of the following exercise program is purposefully designed with specific intentions. It was not by luck or random choice that these exercises are listed in the order they are, but rather by a careful and successfully tested routine that must be followed as shown.

With few exceptions, this program is designed to work the largest muscle groups first, on down through to the smallest groups.

Upper body = Pectorals ---> Deltoids ----> Triceps -----> Biceps ------> Abdominals
           (chest)   (shoulders) (back of arm) (front of arm)   (stomach)

Lower body = Gluteus Maximus ---- > Quadriceps -----> Hamstrings-----> Calves
           (buttocks)   (front of leg)   (back of leg)   (lower leg)

Why, you may ask? What difference does this make? Actually, this type of large muscle to small muscle progression disallows any chance for the targeted parts to fully recuperate, before once again being isolated through another variation of exercise to that same area.

Take your leg exercises, for example. You go from squat, to leg extension, then to leg curl. Although each muscle group is worked in separate fashion, in truth, each muscle exercise *leads into the other.*

A kind of pre-fatiguing signal sent from the larger muscle to the smaller ones ahead as if to say, "better get warmed and ready, because your next." This is another example of how this type of program will typically reduce the number of exercises normally required to do the same job other programs offer. Because overall effectiveness is usually determined more on how smart one works, rather than how *hard.*

IT'S ALL RELATIVE

Finally, one's potential for growth is as largely diversified as all those who exercise. Granted, there are those who are naturally able to develop certain areas, seemingly with little effort. But it should go without saying that more often than not, each respective body part will develop according to the amount of work put into it, plain and simple.

So, if you want big arms and work hard to get them, do not expect your stomach, legs, or any other body part to develop equally without the same focus and attention. Remember, it's all relative!

CHAPTER EIGHT:

WARM-UP

If exercise is now to be a part of your life, you must again prepare yourself. No, not so much on the mental side this time, but more in terms of physical preparedness. That of *warming up*.

Unfortunately, there are many today who still neglect this important step prior to sports and exercise. But a proper warm-up routine plays just as important a role as the exercise program itself. It's not an option!

Take our professional athletes for instance. They recognize the warm-up period as a critical element towards the maintaining and future of their success. Therefore, you should treat it no differently. In fact, it is even more important for you as a non-professional athlete than those who are, regardless of your present fitness level.

The weekend warrior, high school or college athlete, or general all around fitness buff must realize that no one person or group is excused or allowed to bypass warming up before undertaking any form of strenuous physical activity. So don't start picking up those barbells just yet.

WHY?

A person who warms up properly will find their body responding much quicker and easier to the demands put upon it. It also creates an increased capacity for sustained exercise, thus enabling you to excel to your very best while drastically cutting down the chance of injury.

No one welcomes injury, yet, still many believe they are above it. Those who make the habit of taking warming up for granted, more often than not, sooner or later, will find themselves with any one of a possible variety of injuries. Some of the most common are torn or pulled muscles, torn cartilage, back spasms, shin splints, or ankle sprains just to name a few.

Injury to the muscle is not good. Injury to a joint is even worse.

NOT THE SAME THING

Also, the concept of warming up is many times confused with the same thing as stretching. Close but not true. Stretching alone is not considered a proper warm-up. If possible, try to avoid stretching a muscle when it is cold, or in other words, one that has not been properly prepared for sudden or strenuous activity.

One should first engage in some form of non-strenuous activity that *gradually* prepares the muscles, joints, lungs, and heart, *all at the same time*. An activity that will raise the heart rate to a safe, but somewhat moderate level. A short-term activity that will increase the pumping of blood throughout the entire body, in turn, providing you with a loose, warm feeling. Only then should you begin to stretch.

GETTING PRIMED FOR EXERCISE

Before you begin, first consider the questions below before choosing one or more of the following warm-up exercises, then proceed accordingly.

1) Evaluate what kind of sport or activity are you preparing for.
2) Determine at what intensity level you plan to attempt during that activity.
3) Be aware of the body part or parts most intensively used during that activity.
4) Always be aware of what your physical limitations are.

Jogging: Weather permitting, I find this to be my favorite warm-up exercise of all. It tends to stimulate most all of the body's working parts in preparation for an entire range of sporting activities. Jogging closely simulates just about any running or jumping activity you can think of. Jog 3-5 minutes or more until sufficiently warmed up.

Running in Place: If you find it hard to make it outside or have no indoor facility available, softly running in place works well, carrying with it basically the same benefits as jogging.

Aerobic Classes: There are a few who prefer to warm-up by enrolling in aerobic classes. These classes are superb for warming one up sufficiently. They not only emphasize the aerobic aspect, but flexibility training as well. Depending on your personal preference for a warm-up time, you can pop in for a quick 5 or 10 minutes, or remain for the duration of the class.

Jumping Jacks: Most commonly referred to as a calisthenic, jumping jacks have served as a long term standby in various warm-up and elementary exercise programs for years. It can be done anywhere, at anytime, without need of special equipment or facilities. It is simple and nothing new, something each of us has done at one time or another.

Jump Rope: Jumping rope is another excellent exercise for complete body stimulation and raising of the heart rate. It is also beneficial in refining your coordination skills. A simple minute or two is all you will probably need, or probably want. It's a lot tougher than it looks.

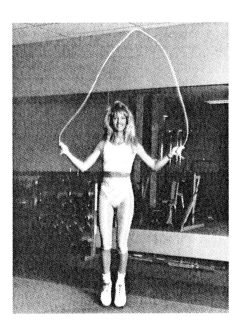

Stationary Bicycle: As further emphasized in chapter 12, "Aerobically Speaking", the stationary bike seems to be the favorite choice of many for warming up before exercise. You should ride until you begin to breathe heavier than normal, and feel close to breaking a sweat. Usually around 3 - 5 minutes.

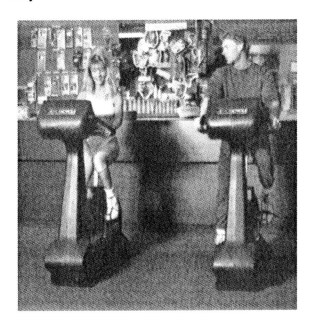

Push Ups: I highly recommend including push ups as part of your warm-up routine if you are preparing to train with weights. This particular exercise is another time-proven standby that is excellent for warming up the major muscles in the upper body and abdomen. It prepares the muscles for the load that will soon be put upon them.

STARTING POSITION:

Lay face down on the floor, head up, and position your hands approximately shoulder-width apart (no wider). Hold your body perfectly straight with the chest lightly touching the floor and feet up on the toes.

STEP 1

Exhale as you push up until the arms are extended, while always maintaining a straight body. (Avoid allowing the elbows to venture too close to your sides)

STEP 2

Inhale as you lower yourself, until your chest *lightly* touches the floor. You should notice that the stomach should be around an inch or two off the floor at this point, thus emphasizing strict form.

Push up and repeat. Do 1 - 3 sets of at least 10 or more until you feel sufficiently warmed up.

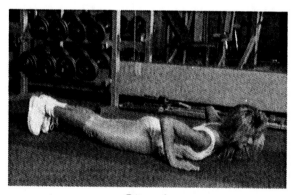

Step 1

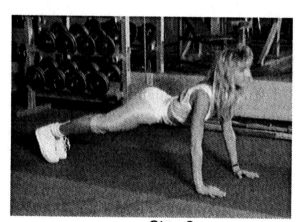

Step 2

***Deep Knee Bends*:** The deep knee bend warm-up can be an excellent exercise by itself, one that closely simulates the squat exercise that you will be doing in a later chapter. It is a basic warm-up exercise for almost any physical activity. It strengthens, stretches, and prepares the various components of your legs for physical exertion.

STARTING POSITION:
Begin standing, with hands on hips and feet slightly narrower than shoulder-width apart, around 12 - 15 inches. (You may want to begin by placing a thick book, or a 2 X 4 piece of wood under your heels, until you gain in flexibility and balance.)

STEP 1
Inhale while lowering yourself all the way down, extending your arms out front to aid in balance.

STEP 2
Focus to a point on a wall in front of you while keeping your head up and back straight, (don't look down). Exhale as you stand back up, bringing your hands back to the hips in starting position. Do 2 - 3 sets of 10 or more until sufficiently warmed up.

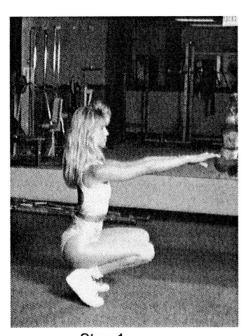
Step 1

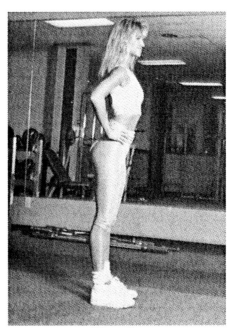
Step 2

STRETCHING SOLO

Now that you have the blood pumping and feel ready to move on, it is now recommended that you pre-stretch the muscle or muscle group you are about to start working. A series of stretching movements should be included in your weight training warm-up routine aimed at matching or *simulating* those same movements that you will be doing for each respective exercise.

Do this; *Analyze the types of exercises about to be performed, then develop a series of stretches on your own for what you feel your body needs.*

Think about it! This is where a little bit of the responsibility is purposely placed upon you. This is your chance to take off those proverbial training wheels and simply experiment. See, feel, experience the different sensations certain stretching positions provide. Find your limits as well as your likes. Take it upon yourself to spark a little self-interest in the learning-by-doing process.

If you need some ideas or examples, refer to the chapter called "Warm-Down" for more of an in-depth guide to some specific stretching practices.

CHAPTER NINE:

GET WITH THE PROGRAM
(Full body Toning, Strength, and Muscle Development)

Hey guys, you want those ripped, well proportioned, defined arms and chest? Perhaps a little tighter stomach area, deflating that old spare tire? And gals, how about a tighter, more toned pair of thighs and buttocks? What about a better defined shoulder and bust line area for enhancing those eye-pleasing curves? Let's also not forget the importance of improved posture and flexibility? And for all you athletes in serious training or those merely under the heading of a weekend warrior, added strength and explosive muscle responsiveness would be a definite bonus, right?

OK, this is it! This is what you have been waiting for. The time to start sculpting yourself a brand new body is here. So lets get out the hammer and chisel and get busy.

Again, honestly assess your present physical condition with respect to your immediate and long-term goals. If your ambitions lean more toward muscle toning, strength, and/or body sculpting, you're in the right place. This will be your *most direct route!* But if the emphasis is more in the direction of fat loss and weight control, chapter twelve should take a little higher priority at this particular time. Seniors and teens, your focus should begin in chapter thirteen, "For All Ages".

At this point, after finally having established an exercise base with the four previous set-up chapters, you should now be adequately prepared to choose from one of the following weight training programs that fit best. Choose carefully and wisely. If you find the beginners program still to be too difficult to start with, choose from a variety of lower intensity exercises given in chapter thirteen called "For All Ages". Remember, always stay within your own physical limits! Now, grab your water bottle and let's get down to it!

BEGINNERS

(3 DAYS PER WEEK)

WARM-UP

1)	SQUAT	1 SET OF 10-15 REPS
2)	LEG EXTENSION	1 SET OF 10-15 REPS
3)	LEG CURL	1 SET OF 10-15 REPS
4)	BENCH PRESS	1 SET OF 8-12 REPS
5)	OVERHEAD PRESS	1 SET OF 8-12 REPS
6)	TRICEP EXTENSION	1 SET OF 8-12 REPS
7)	LAT PULL-DOWN	1 SET OF 8-12 REPS
8)	INCLINE CURL	1 SET OF 8-12 REPS
9)	AB-CROSS BURNOUT	1 SET OF AMAP *

WARM-DOWN

*AMAP (as many as possible)

Monday-Wednesday-Friday
OR
Tuesday-Thursday-Saturday

******************** CAUTION ********************

Before moving on to the next level of intensity, allow plenty of time for your body to become accustomed to the effects of the beginner workout first, then proceed gradually.

****

INTERMEDIATE

(3 DAYS PER WEEK)

WARM-UP

1)	SQUAT	2-3 SETS OF 10-15 REPS
2)	LEG EXTENSION	2-3 SETS OF 10-15 REPS
3)	LEG CURL	2-3 SETS OF 10-15 REPS
4)	BENCH PRESS	2-3 SETS OF 6-12 REPS
5)	HORIZONTAL DUMBBELL FLYE	2-3 SETS OF 6-12 REPS
6)	OVERHEAD PRESS	2-3 SETS OF 6-12 REPS
7)	TRICEP EXTENSION	2-3 SETS OF 6-12 REPS
8)	BENT-OVER ROWING	2-3 SETS OF 6-12 REPS
9)	INCLINE CURL	2-3 SETS OF 6-12 REPS
10)	BENT-KNEE SIT-UP	2-3 SETS OF AMAP *
	and/or	
11)	AB-CROSS BURNOUT	2-3 SETS OF AMAP *
	WARM-DOWN	

* AMAP (as many as possible)

Monday-Wednesday-Friday
OR
Tuesday-Thursday-Saturday

Give yourself at least a couple of months or more before moving on to the advanced sections. If you follow and execute the intermediate program correctly, **you may not have need for anything more,** as in the case for most who will read this book. Remember, a practical and reasonable approach in program selection will play a big part towards long-term success. In other words, if you are comfortable with what is transpiring, stay with it.

But for those who continue to strive for perfection, perhaps desire a higher degree of athletic prowess, or for whatever the rhyme or reason, take it to new heights with this next level of training. *Advanced* training!

Be sure to note that due to the increased number of sets per exercise, the more advanced programs will now emphasize training only half of the body in any one single workout session, rather than the entire body all at once (as in both the beginner and intermediate layout). Quite simply, work the upper body one day and the lower the next.

This will enable you to not only generate maximum intensity during each respective exercise, but more importantly, be able to maintain a sufficient level of energy towards the completion of each given program throughout its entirety. Attempting to perform more than 3 sets on all 14 or so different body part exercises, *all in one training period*, will undoubtedly lead to a running out of gas long before ever reaching the end.

Granted, hard work is what it's all about. But never get out of the habit of working hard AND working equally **efficient** as well.

ADVANCED

(4 DAYS PER WEEK)

LOWER BODY

WARM-UP
1)	SQUAT	3-5 SETS OF 10-15 REPS
2)	LEG EXTENSION	3-5 SETS OF 10-15 REPS
3)	LEG CURL	3-5 SETS OF 10-15 REPS
4)	BENT-KNEE SIT-UP	3 SETS OF AMAP *
	and/or	
5)	AB-CROSS BURNOUT	3 SETS OF AMAP *
	WARM-DOWN	

* AMAP (as many as possible)

Monday-Thursday

UPPER BODY

WARM-UP
1)	BENCH PRESS	3-5 SETS OF 6-12 REPS
2)	HORIZONTAL DUMBBELL FLYE	3-5 SETS OF 6-12 REPS
3)	OVERHEAD PRESS	3-5 SETS OF 6-12 REPS
4)	TRICEP EXTENSION	3-5 SETS OF 6-12 REPS
5)	BENT-OVER ROWING	3-5 SETS OF 6-12 REPS
6)	INCLINE CURL	3-5 SETS OF 6-12 REPS
7)	BENT-KNEE SIT-UP	3-5 SETS OF AMAP *
	and/or	
8)	AB-CROSS BURNOUT	3-5 SETS OF AMAP *
	WARM-DOWN	

*AMAP (as many as possible)

Tuesday-Friday

   If possible, I recommended that you incorporate some sort of aerobic or endurance training either before or after weight training or on the days you are not working with weights. It doesn't have to be much, just something that will further stimulate your cardiovascular and respiratory system.

   Nevertheless, if you follow precisely as instructed, with special emphasis on the amount of time you rest between each set, you shouldn't lack near as much of the aerobic potential as you would in other traditional weight lifting **only** programs. (Refer back to chapter seven, under "Set Intervals".)

OVERLOAD

(6 DAYS PER WEEK)

UPPER BODY

WARM-UP

1)	BENCH PRESS	3-5 SETS OF 6-12 REPS
2)	HORIZONTAL DUMBBELL FLYE	3-5 SETS OF 6-12 REPS
3)	OVERHEAD PRESS	3-5 SETS OF 6-12 REPS
4)	TRICEP EXTENSION	3-5 SETS OF 6-12 REPS
5)	BENT-OVER ROWING	3-5 SETS OF 6-12 REPS
6)	INCLINE CURL	3-5 SETS OF 6-12 REPS
7)	BENT-KNEE SIT-UP	3-5 SETS OF AMAP *
8)	AB-CROSS BURNOUT	3-5 SETS OF AMAP *

WARM-DOWN

*AMAP (as many as possible)

Monday-Wednesday-Friday

LOWER BODY

WARM-UP

1)	SQUAT	3-5 SETS OF 10-15 REPS
2)	LEG EXTENSION	3-5 SETS OF 10-15 REPS
3)	LEG CURL	3-5 SETS OF 10-15 REPS
4)	BENT-KNEE SIT-UP	3 SETS OF AMAP*
5)	AB-CROSS BURNOUT	3 SETS OF AMAP*

WARM-DOWN

* AMAP (as many as possible)

Tuesday-Thursday-Saturday

OVERLOAD

The primary purpose of this next and last program called "Overload", is merely to shock the body a little differently than what it has normally become accustomed to, in an effort to promote further stimulation in growth and development. It works great when additional levels of motivation and desire are present for those few extremists who wish to tackle more.

However, this particular program *should not be attempted by anyone but the die-hard experienced, that carry higher than average goals.* It is also not recommended for those over the age of 35, due to the decline of adequate recuperation time needed by the body as age increases.

Moreover, regardless of your present fitness level, it's strongly suggested that you not undertake this program longer than a month at any one length of time. Again, this should be used only as a short term shocker. Any longer stretch of time may prove to be non-productive, possibly even detrimental. Even if you fail to feel it physically, you will eventually begin to feel it mentally, usually in the form of burnout. So here again, more is not always better.

Instead, design your schedule to incorporate this 6 day per week Overload program only once or twice a year usually in your off-season. Each, for a period of only 1 month maximum, in an effort to keep the body guessing, and yet, allow appropriate time for adequate mind and muscle recuperation.

(I thought this concept was worth mentioning because it worked well for me a few times early on in my training years. Chiefly, at non-specific times when my workout results needed a boost.)

COME ON, LETS GET PUMPED!

*There is NO elevator to success, in **anything**.*
Like everyone else, you too, must first climb the stairs!

As in anything of value worth having, dedication and work are the primary ingredients. Knowing and accepting this is winning half the battle. The other half is doing it. There is no easy way to get in shape or get the results you want. No fads, gimmicks, shortcuts, or sales pitches, can replace or come close to, *good old fashion work*. If that's understood, lets get started!

****

Due to the popularity of upper body development and because 65% of the body's muscles are above the hips, instruction will begin in the order of the Bench Press exercise first. For most, the need for greater upper body strength and definition usually outweigh and take priority over other lower body parts. It does not however, make the lower body any less important.

In whatever program level you may have chosen, Beginner, Intermediate or Advanced, **make sure you follow it**.

If, per chance, you do run into a specific exercise snag, then and only then, will it be time to refer to the section entitled, "Troubleshooting" provided toward the back of this book.

****

BENCH PRESS

The Bench Press is one of the basic, most fundamental strength building exercises used by coaches and athletes since the early days of weight training. It not only emphasizes greater strength, but equally provides a necessary structural and fundamentally sound base as well. It is an essential part of any exercise routine, among one of the most popular.

The Bench Press exercise is excellent for developing upper body mass, more specifically, the pectoral muscles or "pecs" for short. These are more commonly referred to as your chest muscles.

The Bench Press gives men that solid, armor plated look, in contrast to a firmer, more defined bust line in women.

It is a relatively simple exercise with the exception that if you are using a large amount of weight, or unsure of your capabilities, it would be wise to use a spotter for safety reasons. Otherwise, stick to a weight you can handle by yourself as outlined earlier in part by the "M.E.T." concept; "Take It Off."

BODY POSITION

To start, lay flat on your back with feet apart and flat on the floor. You are now in a stable position to support yourself during this exercise. Grasp the bar overhead in a medium-wide grip position as shown (a little wider than shoulder width).

Maintain a firm wrist by resting the bar more on the heel of your hand.

BEGIN

Start by lifting the bar off of the rack to an overhead position.

STEP 1

Slowly and smoothly lower the bar until it lightly touches the nipple area of the chest, (avoid bouncing off the chest).

STEP 2

Next, press the bar upward, thus extending the arms fully (stopping just short of fully locking the elbows).

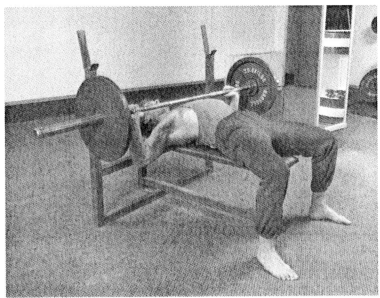
Step 1

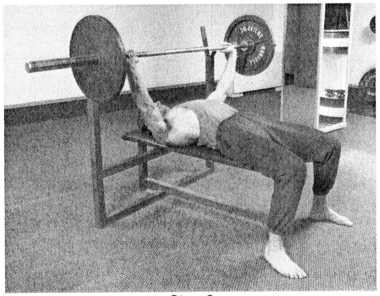
Step 2

******************** IMPORTANT *******************

   To avoid possible injury to the lower back, always keep your buttocks on the bench throughout the entire exercise motion. If you have to strain so hard that your tail end raises up off the bench, you probably have added on too much weight.

****

HORIZONTAL DUMBBELL FLYE

Great! You just finished the Bench Press and have just stimulated those pectorals. You should be satisfactorily warmed up by now. But we are not done with the pecs just yet. This next exercise will put on the finishing touches and accelerate the results you are looking for. That plated, solid look in men, and a more sleek defined look in women.

If you didn't feel as much as you thought you should in the last exercise, you should really feel it in this one. The use of dumbbells in this exercise does a super job in isolating the pectoral muscle group. Here, the targeted area will experience a good pump in the chest, bringing warm feelings of increased blood flow as well as a great stretch of the chest, shoulder, and upper arm muscles. The feeling of the pecs starting to define and tie together will soon follow.

The Horizontal Dumbbell Flye is exactly what the name implies. You are horizontal to the ground, with dumbbell weights for resistance in each hand, working the chest area in sort of a flying or flapping motion. A smooth, yet powerful simulation, similar to an eagle in flight.

Again, I want to stress using very light weight to start with. This is one of those exercises that can be most deceiving, that just when you think you're using light enough weight, in truth, it can still be too much. You will be pleasantly surprised with the feeling you will get by using *too easy a weight* to start with. Only until you acquire the correct motion, rhythm, and feel, should you then proceed to add weight accordingly.

BODY POSITION

Start by first assuming the same position as you did on the Bench Press, on your back with feet on the floor. Grasp one dumbbell in each hand firmly, but not too tight. By over-gripping, you tend to divert your concentration and the overall effectiveness of this exercise.

BEGIN

The starting position is with the dumbbells together, straight over your chest-nipple area with arms extended. Keep the elbows slightly bent to prevent over-stress of the elbow joint.

STEP 1

Gently lower the weights out to your side in a *wide circular motion,* as far out and down as your flexibility will allow while inhaling deeply. Feel the stretch.

STEP 2

Then smoothly, (again in a wide circular motion with arms extended), exhale while raising the dumbbells to arms length over your chest, back to the starting position. Now FLEX those pecs.

Repeat until you have finished the set.

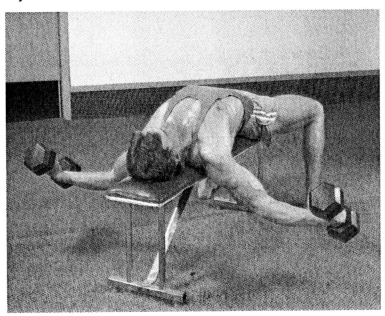

Step 1

Step 2

Do not bang the weights together at the top, at most, allow them to lightly touch at the *same time* you are flexing.

OVERHEAD PRESS

Alright now! You have just completed bombing your chest, which is the largest muscle group in the upper body (with the exception of your back). You should start to feel a pretty good pump by now. With this, you are now ready to tackle the next muscle group in line, the *deltoids*. Others prefer to simply call them the shoulders. There are three basic muscles of the deltoid group consisting of the front, middle, and rear.

The exercising and stimulation of the deltoids, (or delts as the experienced gym-a-holics call them), go hand-in-hand in the forming of that all important base in addition to a powerful chest.

It is common to observe those who take this exercise lightly, or skip this important step altogether, just concerning themselves in the pursuit of building big arms or other eye-pleasing body parts. Actually, it's probably the most neglected area of the body.

A well developed pair of shoulders will not only provide a more structurally balanced body, but actually accentuates the arms even more. They provide that essential, defined look that separates them from the rest of the arms, biceps and triceps.

This must-do exercise goes for people of all ages and professions, not just athletes. Simply put, properly developed shoulders are vital, functionally as well as aesthetically.

BODY POSITION

Assume a sitting position on a flat bench using good posture, back straight, shoulders square, and feet flat on the floor. Grasp the bar with a shoulder-width hand grip, with the bar lightly resting top of your upper chest\collarbone area. You should feel a full stretch of your deltoids while in this position.

BEGIN

The overhead press, commonly called the military press, is another exercise much like the Bench Press, in that its motion is fairly simple.

STEP 1

Push the bar overhead until the arms are fully extended (stopping just before full lock of the elbows).

STEP 2

Lower the bar back to starting position while descending in a controlled manner. Repeat until you finish the set.

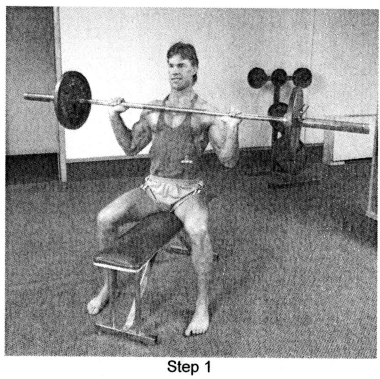

Step 1

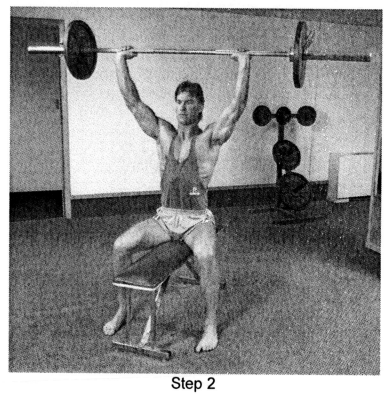

Step 2

******************** IMPORTANT ********************

If you have back problems or are fairly inexperienced in weight training, I suggest you use extra care when first attempting this exercise. Some feel out of balance during the overhead pressing phase without some kind of additional back support. This can lead to undue stress on the lower back or possibly even falling.

The best suggestion I can make is to use lighter weight or find a spotter. Find a friend or someone that can spot you during this exercise, aiding you in the tough spots and thus preventing any mishaps.

If you are lucky enough to have access to specialized apparatus, such as an upright bench solely made for this exercise, by all means use it. Especially at first. It ensures a much safer exercise and ease of learning.

While some use spotters or specialized benches, others compensate by growing entirely dependent on lifting belts for support. If at first you feel better using one, go ahead. But know that little support is gained and you should learn not to depend on this type of training tool too heavily (refer back to chapter six under exercise equipment).

****

TRICEP EXTENSION

This next exercise called the Tricep Extension will emphasize the direct stimulation of the triceps. They are the three muscles that wrap around the back of the arm between the elbow and shoulder. The proper development of this muscle group will make up most of the upper arm mass in men, while giving women that sleek, defined appearance to the arm, in contrast to the baggy look.

The importance of the tricep muscle group here is, that they are not only required to complete the look, but are an essential part of the combined strength effort of the chest, shoulders and back. Without proper development here, the rest of the muscles of the upper body would be of little use.

Working the tricep muscles at this particular time in the program also conforms to our concept of working *the largest muscles down to the smallest*, thus disallowing any unnecessary recuperation. This in turn, will drastically save a lot of extra time and effort from having to re-fatigue the same muscle all over again.

Think about it! Your triceps have just received an indirect stimulation along with a certain amount of fatigue during the first three exercises. In other words, they were being used, but not emphasized. Now, it is their turn to be *isolated*.

Why go off and work your biceps or legs for example, then come back later after the triceps have fully recuperated? It just wouldn't make sense. Isn't the primary purpose to fatigue the muscle in the first place, **in the most efficient way possible?**

Hopefully, with a little experience you will begin to understand why each respective exercise is placed where it is.

BODY POSITION

I recommend using the back pull down machine (or something similar) in a standing position as shown in the following photos in order to achieve maximum effect. If you fail to have access to such apparatus, proceed on further in this chapter to the alternative tricep exercise that requires only a bench.

Otherwise, stay with this standing approach as a first choice. If done correctly, it will result in faster, more efficient gains.

Standing in an upright position, and with a slight inward lean, you should maintain a hand grip approximately shoulder-width apart. The placement of the feet should be rather narrow, with one foot or the other placed slightly ahead of the other to ensure better overall balance and isolation of the exercise.

BEGIN
   The starting position is with the elbows close to the side and with the bar across the chest. Each repetition must begin from a complete stop. No swinging, bouncing, or jerking.

STEP 1
   While maintaining the position of the elbows at your side, extend the arms downward in an outward circular motion until the arms become fully extended.

STEP 2
   In the same outward circular motion, gently allow the arms to bend back upward into starting position. Repeat until you have finished the set.

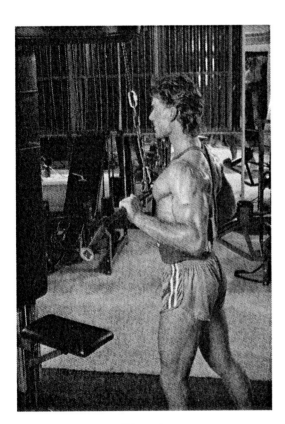

Step 1

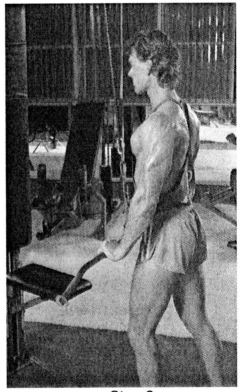

Step 2

Alternative Selection to the standing Tricep Extension

TRICEP EXTENSION
on a bench

BODY POSITION
Assume a flat position on your back with feet apart on the floor to aid in balance. Your head should be hanging just off the end of the bench.

BEGIN
Starting position is with the bar <u>over the head</u>, not the chest. The hand grip should be slightly narrower than shoulder-width.

STEP 1
In a wide, reverse circular motion, gently bend at the elbows and lower the bar down to the forehead. Here, the forearm is the only thing that should move.

STEP 2
Again, without rotating anything but the forearm and in an outward circular motion, extend the arms fully back to starting position.

I caution you to be extra careful when lowering the bar so as not to bang your forehead. Also, keep the buttocks on the bench at all times.

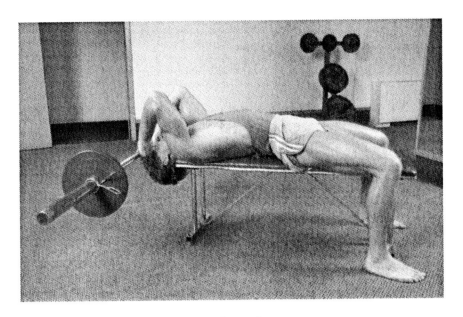

Step 1

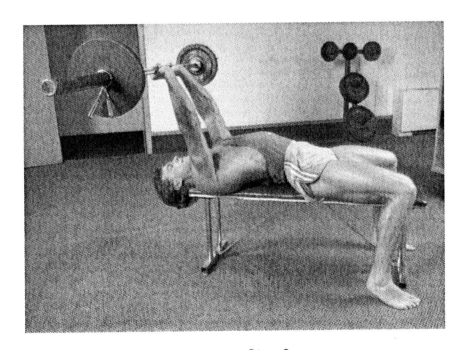

Step 2

BENT-OVER ROWING

****************** CAUTION *******************

This particular exercise should be omitted by ALL individuals, except those who fall into any one of the following categories below;

- Only athletes in training
- Only those with no history of back problems.
- Only those in moderate to excellent physical shape and show good flexibility.

Although, this is probably the riskiest back exercise one can do, it is also one of the most productive. Simply stay within your physical limits and exercise sensibly.

For everyone else, I recommend an alternative exercise such as the Lat Pull-Down machine as shown further along in this chapter.

****

OUT OF ORDER?

Up to this point we have succeeded in the stimulation and fatiguing of the chest, shoulders, and part of the upper arms respectively, thus keeping with concept of working the larger muscles on down to the smaller ones, except for now.

At this point, and only at this point of our upper body program, will we temporarily step out of our *largest to smallest* order of exercises, and work the back, the largest combined muscle group in the upper body.

What, you may ask, is the reasoning behind this? Up to now things were just beginning to make sense. Well, hang in there and try not to get confused.

Theoretically, the back should have been the very first exercise completed in a typical upper body workout, primarily because of size alone. But experience has shown that the back is still not adequately warmed up at that early stage, making injury highly probable.

Instead, you will find that at this particular point in the program, the back is more apt to be stretched and ready for the exertion it will be forced to undergo. In addition, this exercise has a tendency to pre-fatigue the bicep muscle in preparation for the next exercise in the program. So, buckle up and shift gears to one of the most important areas of our musculature system, the back.

The Bent-Over Rowing exercise will develop the side Lat and back muscles, mainly those which make up the outside and lower portions of the back. It will give men that wide "V" shaped look, while helping women attain that long, sought after, hourglass shape. This exercise will not only add thickness and strength, but help maintain lower back flexibility as well.

Again, athletes recognize the importance of a strong back, and so should you. Without it, there would be little support for all that is required, whether engaging in various sporting activities, or simply surviving the common efforts of everyday life.

You say you have back problems. Well, as it turns out, roughly 80% of those experiencing lower back problems have been caused by muscular weakness in that area brought about by sedentary lifestyles. Neglecting the problem will not make it go away! All in all, proper back flexibility and strength training is essential for any and all, towards maintaining a functionally synchronized and well balanced upper body.

BODY POSITION

Assume a bent over position, an angle somewhere between 45 and 90 degrees, back straight, and head up. The feet should be no wider than shoulder-width with the knees slightly bent. (The bent knees aid one in flexibility and cut down on lower back stress.)

BEGIN

Start by gripping the bar with the hands together in the middle of the bar, with not more than a few inches between them. Pick up the bar, allowing it to hang naturally from the arms.

(For some, this may feel a little uncomfortable at first due to the certain degree of balance required, but do it anyway. Learn to acquire a feel for it.)

The exercise motion itself is much the same to that of rowing a boat, from which the name was taken.

STEP 1

Starting from a dead hang, pull the bar up until your wrists touch the hip bone area, not the stomach or the legs, but the point at where your body bends.

STEP 2

In a controlled manner, gently lower the bar until the arms are once again fully extended. Repeat this procedure until you have finished the set.

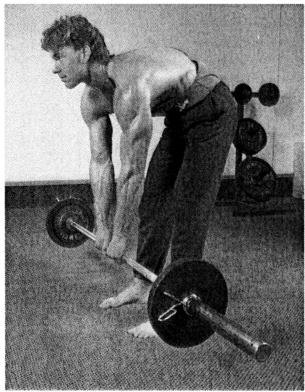

Step 1

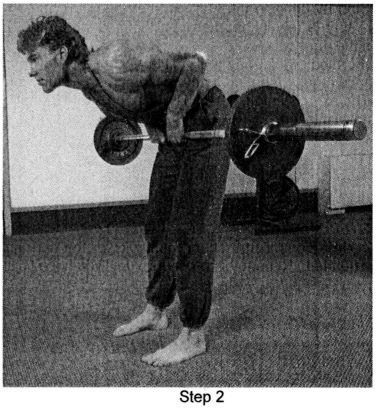

Step 2

There are other methods of doing this exercise, but greater overall results will be found at this time by doing it in a close-grip fashion. It tends to stimulate the entire range of the lat muscle **at one time**, rather than breaking it up into strictly upper or lower back exercises as in some of the traditional wider grips. Again, this lessens the overall exercise time frame and increases efficiency.

******************** Helpful Hint ********************

A very effective alternative to using a straight bar would be a "T-bar" apparatus or a specifically designed "rowing bench". Unfortunately, these types of apparatus are not all that common.

****

Alternative Selection To Bent-Over Rowing

LAT PULL-DOWN

The Lat Pull-Down is a much safer exercise in regard to the lower back. The degree of stress is greatly reduced, while the degree of effectiveness is decreased only slightly.

For this exercise you must have access to some kind of Pull-Down apparatus like the one shown in the given illustrations.

BODY POSITION

The most popular type of pull down machines, are those that you sit facing the machine with bar hanging overhead. If this is what you are using, position yourself so that your knees are tucked securely under the given restraining pads, if so equipped. These will keep you from lifting yourself out of position during the lift. If there are no such pads, use lighter resistance.

Certain other machines such as "Nautilus", dictate that you face away from the machine and feature an adjustable seat and a securing strap, such as the one illustrated. If so, adjust the seat so that when you grip the bar overhead you are in a fully stretched position. At this point the weights should be just slightly off the rack.

BEGIN

A popular method of executing this exercise is usually done by using a very wide hand grip, pulling the bar down until it touches the back of the neck. This is a good exercise and a standard in many programs. But most who try it usually find faster results by this other method:

Regardless of the style of machine, begin by gripping the bar overhead with a reversed hand grip (palms facing you) as if you were going to do a chin-up. The hands should be fairly close to each other in the center of the bar.

STEP 1

From a fully extended and stretched position, pull the bar down and touch the upper chest area.

STEP 2

Allow the bar to return back up to stretched position, but always in a controlled manner. Repeat until you finish the set.

116

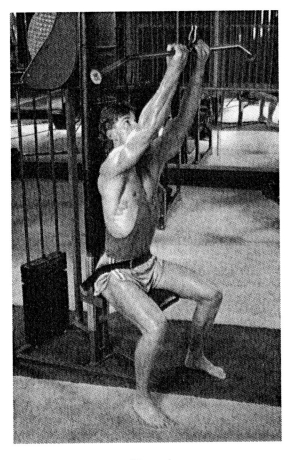

Step 1

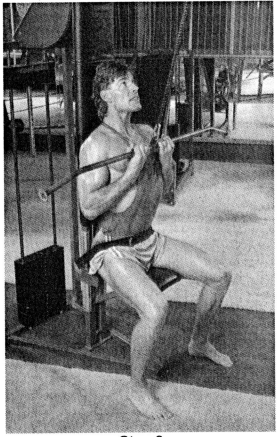

Step 2

INCLINE CURL

It is now time to get back to the prescribed order of working the *largest to the smallest* muscle groups. This comes after briefly stepping out of line with the previous Bent Over Rowing exercise, and continue on with the next exercise called, the Incline Curl.

This particular weight training exercise is one of the biggest eye-opening, physically stimulating ones that you can do. You will feel the results almost immediately, and be able to see them nearly as fast. *If done correctly*, it will not only inspire and motivate, but also play a significant role in building confidence in the program as well. It will simply PUMP..... YOU..... UP!

The method of instruction and execution of this next exercise will shorten the time frame by *at least* a third of the time it normally takes one to notice results from doing other related exercises. The Incline Curl will be the turning point for those who have unsuccessfully searched, strained, and labored, in the quest of acquiring a toned, well developed bicep.

DREAMING OF THE DAY

For many, the popularity and importance of working the bicep muscle seems to overshadow just about all other areas of interest. This is especially true regarding to the male gender.

Ever since childhood young boys have stood in front of the mirror flexing their biceps, dreaming of a day when they would pop through their shirt. It still holds true today, in homes and gyms all across the country. He, who once was a boy, is now a man. This same individual, along with thousands like him, are still trying to get that long awaited, bulging bicep. They continue to grunt, swing, jerk and curl weights for months, even years on end with little to show for their efforts, until now.

Females, alike, will benefit much in the same way by doing this exercise, but more along the lines of more fit and finer toned arms.

But before moving on, let us not stray from the more important reasons for developing a good bicep. It is here I re-emphasize the importance of increased strength, flexibility, and functional capabilities. Remember, one that looks good, should also work, as well.

BODY POSITION

This exercise requires a bench with a back support inclined on an angle somewhere around 45 degrees. Many times these particular benches are adjustable merely by inserting or pulling a pin.

Sit with your back flat against the back support. Feet should be flat on the floor in a support position as shown.

118

BEGIN

Keep the shoulders square and back against the bench while allowing the arms to hang straight down. Maintain position of the dumbbells as shown in step 1 and step 2 throughout the entire motion. Do not turn or twist the wrists at this time.

STEP 1

Beginning from a dead hang and with the arms limp, curl the dumbbells up simultaneously, until they touch the **side** of the lower chest area.

STEP 2

Next, uncoil the biceps by gently lowering the dumbbells until the arms have reached full extension down next to your side. You should now feel a good STRETCH. Repeat until the set is finished.

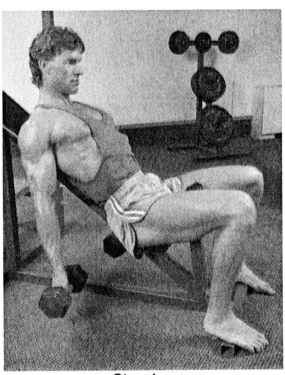

Step 1

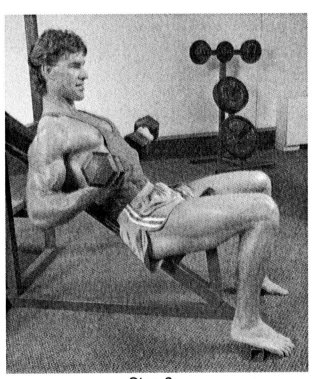

Step 2

There are some who prefer to alternate arms during this exercise. But experience has shown that alternating from one arm to another negatively effects one's overall technique.

It allows the body position to shift, even if it's only a little, along with a tendency to swing the dumbbells up, rather than a strict curling motion. There are very few individuals who can do this without breaking form and/or concentration in some way or another.

There are those who will dispute this, and there are others who will find that it does work better. But I urge you to stay on the outlined path as given, thus keeping things simple and productive.

BENT-KNEE SIT-UP

We are now at a point in the program at which I believe to be the prime indicator in which good health and physical condition are judged, especially in men. That's right, I am referring to the abdominal region (abs for short), more commonly remembered as your stomach muscles.

Next time you are at the gym or in a club atmosphere, look around and take time to notice how many so-called exercise buffs, actually stress the importance of working their abdominals as much as they do their biceps, chest, or any other upper body part. And if they do participate in a few sit-ups, how serious are they? Look and judge for yourself, it isn't hard to figure out.

Despite why some do, and why many more don't, the proper development of the abdominal muscles are probably more important than any other muscle group in the body. They become the focal point and driving force from which most all movement is initiated. They are also responsible for maintaining proper body alignment and back support. All in all, they happen to be yet another essential component in providing that ever-so-important structural and fundamentally sound base.

Besides, any person with a flat, well defined stomach region not only looks good, but probably is lower in body fat, and experiences fewer digestive problems. Women, on the other hand, tend to desire a flat tummy for other reasons in addition to the ones just mentioned. One that comes to mind, is the after-effects of having children, a definite need to re-tighten that particular area.

Therefore, the objective of this exercise is to tighten, define, and further develop the muscles of the *entire* abdominal region. Sit-ups will increase one's abdominal and back strength, flexibility, and range of motion.

But you must go back and remember, the act of doing sit-ups will not directly help lose fat or deflate a spare tire. It is not possible to *spot reduce* in any one specific area. Fat loss is the result of aerobic exercise combined with a proper diet program. (See Chapter 12, "Aerobically Speaking".)

I doubt there is anyone who has not performed a sit-up at one time in their life, and I understand the awkward and uncomfortable feelings that usually go along with this type of exercise. After all, those feelings of blood rushing to the head, the crunching up of the midsection and a lot of over-exerted effort can be quite a deterrent. But that's mainly what exercise is all about, right?

I guess what it all comes down to is most people would rather feel fatigued in the bicep or thigh area for instance, before they push themselves beyond the comfort zone in their abs. In short, pushing the abs down a little too far on one's priority list.

For others, it may be something else. Perhaps it's fear that scares some away. Fear of something they have either read, heard, experienced, or have been taught. Such as, the effect sit-ups can possibly have on the back, especially those with lower back problems or those seriously overweight.

Actually, their concern is genuine and should always be addressed properly. Most experts in the field of exercise physiology tend to agree, that the Full Sit-Up is another one of those risky exercises that contain the possibility of injury and regard it as something that is and should be a thing of the past.

Granted, continued questioning of one's own potential for injury should always be utmost in one's mind, but more often than not, most of us have proven that it's easier to turn legitimate questions into convenient excuses.

Although the risk factor is present, it is also true that there can be little hope of successfully developing the *entire* abdominal muscle range, without the full and direct stimulation in which the full sit-up exercise provides. Few other, all-in-one, tummy exercises have the ability to *tie in* and synchronize the upper torso directly to the lower torso, and everything in between like the Full Sit-up.

YOU MUST CHOOSE

Agreed, there are numerous other variations to the sit-up, each with its own unique advantages and place in a workout program. But at this time I want the reader to stay within the main objective of this book, in keeping things simple and successful, yet eliminate extra work and time consuming steps. Therefore, you are hereby provided with the two most effective options, each dependent upon your current physical condition and/or limitations.

The first choice is one which we have just referred to, the traditionally sound, Full Sit-Up. Only those who categorize themselves as potential risks to back injury, or are moderately to largely overweight, should overlook this first choice and proceed to the next option called, Ab-Cross burnout. Again, be 100% honest in your personal assessment by following the direction of your conscience. If there are any legitimate doubts, stick with the second option.

But for most of you with no justifiable excuses, and you know who you are, give yourself a chance and try this first exercise precisely the way it is instructed. Forget the way you had to do it in high school P.E. class. This version is much more precise, more defined, thus more profitable in both the long and short run.

This particular technique of a common Sit-Up will, once again, adhere to the time-rendered basic exercise principals that require nothing short of a full range of execution, meaning all the way up, and all the way back down. Too many others would rather do "crunches", (the act of only going part way down on each repetition) either in an honest attempt to isolate a specific abdominal group, or because they usually find them easier to do. Although "crunches" do have their place in certain programs, most continue to do them simply because they are easier. Reality check; crunches and half-way's just won't do it!

A HIGH-REP EXERCISE

In contrast to our set program standard of 6-12 reps per set, you will also find that the abdominal region will respond greater to those sets that involve higher repetitions, rather than worrying too much about resistance. In short, do as many as you can during each set, but only as long as you are able execute correctly without over-straining.

Besides being a high-rep exercise, it is also one that can be done everyday. This is unlike most of the larger muscle groups that require a longer recuperation time. Therefore, I recommend some kind of ab work every day for all athletes or anyone with the desire for perfection. High reps combined with perfect technique every day, will provide you with sensational cuts and definition.

BODY POSITION

I encourage all who attempt this, regardless of how good you think your physical condition is, to position the sit-up board flat on the floor in the beginning. Too many jump right into their sit-up routine on too steep an angle and end up cheating themselves on form as well effectiveness. Many believe the harder it is to do, the faster they will see results. Wrong!

ONLY when you find the exercise motion to be overly easy, should you then increase the angle a little at a time.

Hook your feet under the ankle straps or leg anchors in a 45 degree, bent-knee position as illustrated. The purpose of bending the knees is to eliminate as much lower back stress as possible, while at the same time, further isolate the abs during the exercise movement.

If you do not have access to a sit-up board, lay flat on the floor with your feet anchored under some heavy object such as a bed or couch. You can roll up a towel or blanket for use as a pad over the feet for further comfort and stability.

BEGIN

Loosely interlock your fingers behind the head and assume a stretched out and somewhat rested position. (Or better yet, lightly touch your temples with outstretched fingers and keep them there. This keeps you from pulling or jerking the head.)

STEP 1

Tuck your chin down against the collarbone and **tense the ab muscles first,** then smoothly COIL yourself to the up position. (Do not jerk) Once there, cross the elbow over and touch the opposite knee. If you can't touch the knee, do the best you can.

STEP 2

UNCOIL yourself gently back down into the starting position, with emphasis placed on abdominal control of the descent. Repeat as many times as possible.

DO NOT permit yourself to simply *fall* back down after reaching the top. ALWAYS maintain constant control throughout the entire motion, forcing the *abs* to let you down, not gravity.

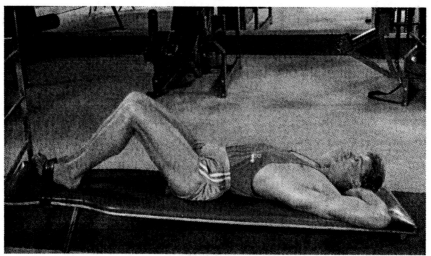

Step1

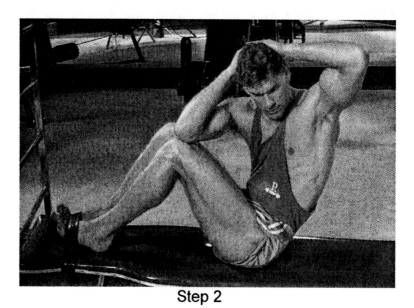

Step 2

******************** Helpful Hint ********************

Many times I find that when trying to teach or explain a certain concept or exercise, as in this case, the substitution of a **"key"** word would make all the difference to something going off in your brain saying, THAT'S IT, I'VE GOT IT!

If you so choose, replace "coil" with words like "ROLL, CRUNCH, or COMPRESS". The word "Uncoil" can replaced by "UNROLL".

****

Although this looks and seems to be a rather easy exercise, do not be surprised to find it to require a certain amount of patience and practice in order to achieve the desired effect.

Alternative and/or Additional Selection To Bent-Knee Sit-Ups

AB-CROSS BURNOUT

For those of you who have been re-directed from the previous sit up exercise to this one, whatever your reasoning may be, the Ab-Cross Burnout is for you. Don't let the name intimidate you. It is an exercise that can be taken to whichever intensity level or goal you so choose, easy or hard.

The Ab-Cross Burnout is another high-rep exercise that directly stimulates the entire abdominal region. It produces much of the same advantages and results as in the Full Sit-Up exercise explained previously. However, it also contains three distinct factors that seem to work well either in addition to the Full Sit-Up, or strictly by itself.

The first, is the ability to experience an incredible burn of each and every abdominal muscle. You can almost feel the separation and defining process transpire. It is an excellent addition to any abdominal exercise program, enabling you to give the abs that finished appearance.

Second, it will allow beginners as well as those who are overweight and out of shape, to learn and familiarize oneself with the different feelings and sensations of what is involved when it comes to working their abs. It is one which almost anyone can do.

Last, but probably the most important reason to include this exercise, is the safety factor. The manner in which this exercise is executed, significantly reduces the chance of injury by keeping the lower back flat on the floor.

BEGINNERS

For the beginner, I insist you try this exercise, knowing full well that it may very well require a certain degree of patience in order to perfect the technique. It is not uncommon to find that timing and coordination play important parts in successfully mastering this particular exercise motion.

Take it at your own speed and hang in there, it WILL be worth the effort.

EXPERIENCED

Those of you who are familiar with this exercise or ones like it, will find it even more productive when incorporating it into your program **immediately after** the Full Sit-Up, or, if you still prefer, simply as an exercise by itself.

I say it again, immediately afterwards. When the mood arises and motivation cries out for more, give it what it wants by blending both exercises together into one set.

For example, as soon as you complete a good set of Sit-Ups and without resting, switch over onto the floor and do as many of the Ab-Crosses as possible, until the abs cease to function. That would count as one set. Do the same for the second set, third set, and so on.

This order of exercise is designed to complete the most difficult one first (Full Sit-Up), then further exhausting the same area by doing the less strenuous one last (Ab-Cross Burnout). Although this routine works extremely well, I advise it only to those experienced or well conditioned individuals, who are considered above average in this particular area.

BODY POSITION

Lie flat on your back, feet together, and hands locked behind your head. You should be in a fully stretched position with both the back of your head and heels of your feet lightly touching the floor.

STEP 1

Begin the first part of the coiling process by tucking the chin down against the center of the collar bone.

Then compress the abdominal muscles in an effort to lift your shoulders just ever so slightly off the floor, while at the same time crossing the elbow over and **aggressively** touching the opposite knee as shown.

Step 1

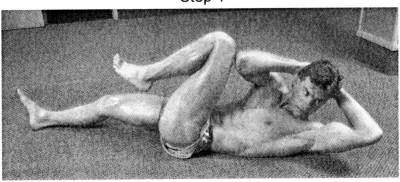

STEP 2

Uncoil the abs and return back to starting position with head back and eyes looking straight up.

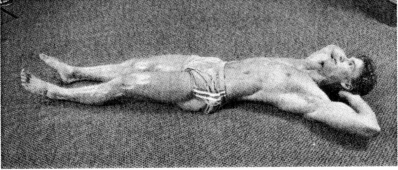

Step 2

127

STEP 3

Tense the abs up again and hit the other knee this time. Repeat each step as many times as possible while continuing to alternate each elbow to the opposite knee.

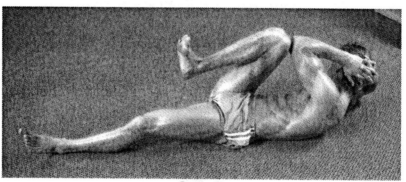

Step 3

Do not try to sit all the way up. Only the shoulders and extreme upper back should raise up, while keeping the lower back pressed firmly against the floor.

THE SQUAT

Squat exercises have much in common with the abdominal exercises as discussed in the previous chapter in respect to being low on one's priority list. This, along with the development of the rest of the lower body, are areas that must be addressed with the same dedication and proper attention as given to the various upper body exercises.

CAUSE FOR CONCERN

"Squatting" has traditionally been met by countless arguments and criticism. Excuses seem to abound why one should not do squats. The most frequent reasons are injury related, and does, in fact, carry a certain amount of credibility with them. It is true that if done in a reckless or incorrect fashion, or in conjunction with certain health or physical limitations, the Squat could prove to be detrimental and unsafe.

Moreover, many orthopedic surgeons have also questioned the advantages versus the risks involved. The risk referred to here is basically in the knee joint. What exercises can you do and how far can you go?

Unless otherwise instructed, the standard to remember here is this;

It is widely recommended not to undertake FULL Squats (sitting all the way down) when lifting heavy amounts of weight, that which would be considered out of the ordinary for your strength capability or present activity level. Instead, only go partial or three quarters of the way down using light to moderate resistance.

However, the overall advantages sometimes out-weigh the disadvantages and should be evaluated fairly and completely before omitting. Those of you who feel unsure of your capabilities should have already checked with your doctor before starting this program.

BEST ALL-AROUND EXERCISE

Basically, the Squat is one of the best exercises one can do to develop the quadriceps or quads for short. (You may commonly refer to them as the thigh region.) It is another exercise much like the Bench Press, in which standards of strength are measured.

Add this to also having a direct and indirect strengthening effect for not only the rest of the leg, but the *entire body as well*. It has been highly acclaimed to be the single most productive barbell exercise one can do. It provides you with a greater sense of balance, body control, and an increased endurance level that's hard to beat.

The unbelievable effect upon the body's metabolism and cardiovascular system will no doubt leave you with a much broader perspective of just what Squats have to offer. Consequently, they carry with them a respectable degree of importance that excludes no one who is capable of undergoing this type of exercise movement.

USE SAFETY EQUIPMENT

For starters, I insist you gain access to some sort of a squat rack or spotting apparatus, similar to the one in the illustration. It provides a much safer exercise and should be used anytime when using any amount of weight.

For those who don't have access to one, I recommend using a fixed-position Leg Sled or Leg Press machine. If these are not available, use zero resistance. Use only a straight bar or broom handle to aid you in body positioning and balance. Then follow the same procedure as per instructed.

*************** VERY IMPORTANT ***************

This is an exercise like no other in regard to starting with too much weight. If you overdo any other exercise by stacking on the weights and pumping out reps, you will no doubt, be understandably stiff and sore afterwards.

BUT, if you overdo this particular exercise too quickly, rather than through a gradual continuation, you will find out first-hand what set-back, pain, and inconvenience is, **the hard way.** If not on the first set, definitely on the second and third. The muscles of the quadriceps, hamstring, glutes, and groin area, all require an explicit warm up and stretching period prior to the first set of squats.

If you completely disregard caution and are lucky enough to avoid serious injury in the process, the painful experience of strained and stretched muscles in the lower torso will, without doubt, remind you every time you move for the next several days.

With this in mind, I recommend **everyone**, regardless of condition, to begin with a straight bar only and no weight. Learn the technique first. Get to know the feeling and balance required before making things more difficult. You will be amazed at how in touch and stimulated one can be, simply by using zero resistance.

****

BODY POSITION

Start from a standing position with the bar (or broom handle) resting across the *back* of your shoulders, not <u>on the neck</u>. Position your elbows so that they are pointing out and slightly back. This will help in keeping the bar as far to the back of the shoulders as possible in an effort to keep the weight centered in a straight line over the body's center of gravity during the entire lift.

This will reduce the need to over-compensate for any forward shifting in balance, in turn, reducing the chances of lower back strain and spinal injury.

Start by gripping the bar fairly wide, to a point where it feels most comfortable with feet positioned around shoulder-width apart. In the beginning, I recommend standing on a 2 X 4 board placed directly under the heels of your feet. If a board is not available, place a couple of the iron barbell plates down on the floor in accordance to your stance, preferably the 25 pounders or larger. A couple of large books work well also. This will aid in further targeting the thigh muscle while increasing control and balance.

(After considerable practice, convert to using NO help from anything under the heels. Instead, learn to squat in a free-form fashion.)

BEGIN

Lift the bar off the rack and assume a standing position. Look up and find a focal point on the ceiling or upper wall.

Next, and this is very important, **LOCK** your back by forming a tight reverse arch, while at the same time sticking the buttocks out as shown. This is done for two important reasons.

The first, is to further ensure the bar remains over your center of gravity. Second, but most importantly, it positions the spine in a more solid and stable position, enabling it to withstand those compressional forces that go with the squat exercise, thus further decreasing the chance of spinal injury.

One more time;

- Keep the head up and focused above.
- Tightly arch the your back in a locked position.
- Execute the lift.

STEP 1

Carefully lower yourself until the thighs are roughly parallel to the ground (or until the legs are bent on a 90 degree angle).
Come to a short, but complete stop. DO NOT bounce at the bottom end.

STEP 2

Keep the head up and push powerfully upward thus extending the legs. You should finish in the same position from which you started. Head up, back tightly arched *and buttocks out.*

Repeat until you have finished the set.

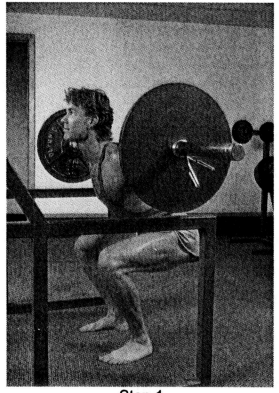
Step 1

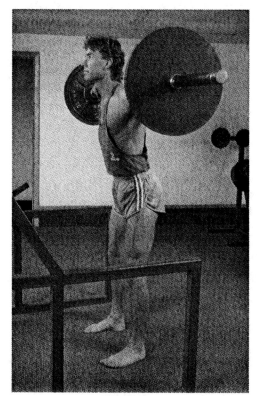
Step 2

Because of the intense cardiovascular activity, it is crucial that proper breathing technique is used. Inhale deeply as you lower yourself, then exhale as you extend upward.

******************** Helpful Hint ********************

If you prefer, as other beginners do, use a chair or bench placed directly behind and underneath you to use as an indicator in letting you know when you have gone down far enough. In other words, you squat down until your rear end lightly touches (do not sit completely), then back up you go again.

This idea is also good for safety reasons. It will help prevent you from falling in case you are unable to stand back up.

****

Again, <u>never bounce off the bottom</u> in the attempt to use momentum to aid you in popping up. This way of thinking is similar to the clutch on your car. If you continue to pop the clutch out too quickly, you will soon find it in the mechanic's shop. The same goes with your knees, only you will require a different kind of mechanic, in a different kind of shop.

But all things considered, I think you will find that the Squat exercise, if performed properly, is probably the hardest one you can do, but in the same respect, is also probably **the most productive one you can do.**

LEG EXTENSION

With the exception of the squat, the Leg Extension is probably one of the best exercises for the development of the upper leg. However, it will primarily focus directly upon the frontal thigh area (quadriceps or quads for short), thus promoting further muscle separation and giving one that complete, defined look.

The knees are also significantly strengthened throughout this exercise. An area critical to everyone's mobility.

This has proven to be a popular leg exercise not only because of the benefits expressed above, but because it turns out to be a more natural and comfortable position in which to exercise. It is one most anyone can do, even those considered out of shape.

BODY POSITION

Sit in an upright position as if you were sitting in any chair. If it has a back rest, use it. If not, maintain proper posture with back straight and shoulders square. Your ankles should be positioned behind the pads with the instep of your feet underneath.

Some Leg Extension apparatus provides you with a hand grip, if so, use it. If not, firmly grasp the side of the bench for additional support.

STEP 1

Beginning from a dead stop, extend the legs fully.

STEP 2

After extending the legs out as far as possible, slowly lower them back to starting position until the weights on the rack *barely touch*, then without resting, extend upward again, repeating both steps over and over until you have finished the set.

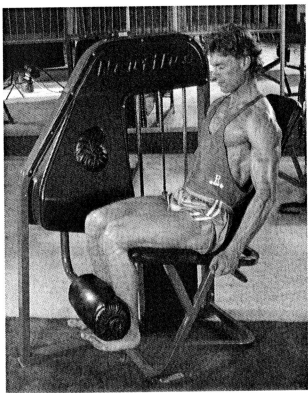

Step 1

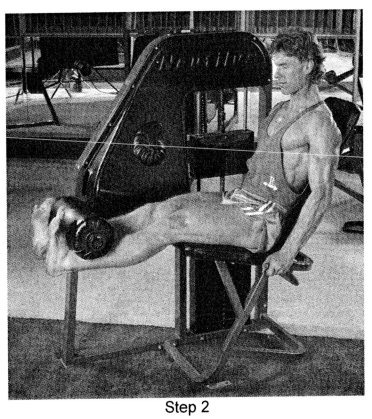

Step 2

LEG CURL

The Leg Curl exercise will directly affect those muscles in the back of your thighs, called the hamstrings. You can think of them as the biceps of your legs. They function opposite the quadriceps, and yet, both work together in order to achieve normal leg movement.

Although the hamstrings are somewhat worked indirectly during the Squat exercise, they still require a need of direct stimulation by way of strict and isolated movements. Here, it is just as important to maintain proper strength equilibrium between the frontal and rear muscles of the thigh as it is in the various muscle groups of the upper body.

If done correctly, the exercise motion of the Leg Curl will not only provide one with a properly developed and functional pair of hamstrings, but will also tie in and stimulate the muscles of the buttocks (gluteus maximus). Still a problem area for millions of Americans today.

*************** A WORD OF CAUTION ***************

If you are to get the most out of this exercise, there are two things you should know first and be aware of:

The first and probably most important is that this exercise, in particular, is another one that is quite deceiving in the sense that it becomes very easy to begin with too much weight. By selecting an easier amount of resistance to begin with, your chances of cheating and using poor technique will greatly diminish, providing speedier results.

The second reason for carefully regulating the resistance is more common sense related, and that is, reducing the chance of injury. When too much weight is used there is a tendency to raise the midsection off the bench and over-stress the lower back.

In addition, the fatiguing of the hamstring muscle has a tendency to sneak up on you. Just when you think you are going along fine, then whammo, your legs are shot. You can really feel it afterwards if you try to bend over and touch your toes.

Overall, this is not a difficult exercise to do, but there are times it could be a little touchy at first.

****

136

BODY POSITION
This exercise will require access to a leg curl machine or a similar apparatus.

Lie on your stomach and hook the backs of your heels under the foot pads (or lower calf area, depending upon your height). Your knees should be positioned just off the edge of the bench. This correctly aligns the knee joint with the rotational axis of the machine.

If the bench is equipped with hand grips, use them. If not, hold on lightly to the sides for additional support.

BEGIN
Always keep your head down and midsection pressed down onto the bench.

STEP 1
Curl your legs up and try to make your heels touch your buttocks, but keep the rear end down.

STEP 2
Gently, and always in a controlled manner, allow the hamstrings to lower the resistance back to the fully extended position, until the weights *lightly touch* (DO NOT bang them at the bottom). Then, without resting, repeat both steps, over and over until the set is finished.

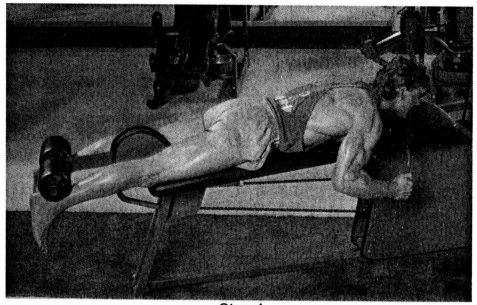

Step 1

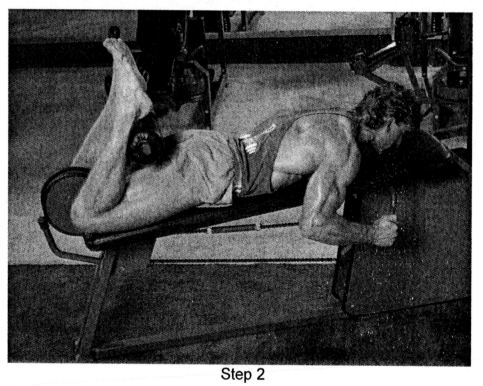

Step 2

CHAPTER TEN:

EXTRA! EXTRA!

Up to now, you have given your body a pretty good workout and may not feel the need to go any further. If that is your choice,then you should feel good about what you have accomplished and work to maintain it. Give yourself a big pat on the back.

However, if you are a serious athlete, or simply one who desires more options, continue on with the following five additional exercises. Through careful thought and consideration, I chose to exclude them from the main exercise program listing itself, chiefly because of my hesitancy to avoid bombarding the reader with too many specialized exercises. My overall intention is to keep the combined number of exercises to a **reasonable** and non-intimidating level, but at the same time, provide one with the option to do more. Because for many, the ability to come away from each workout with that personal sense of fulfillment, can be the most important step toward staying in the fitness game. Especially with regard to such common problem areas as our waistline and buttocks. Only when one begins to actually see and feel such positive things happening to their body, is the likelihood of failure pushed further and further away.

Read on through this chapter and decide for yourself if any one of these exercise options fit into your pre-set goals or desired intensity levels. Although you have been given a choice, I do encourage most to give at least one or two a try.

Toward the end of this chapter is a listing of where the following exercises should fit in if you were to add them to your main program.

LUNGES

(OPTIONAL)

The Lunge is an exercise many feel unnecessary or not worth adding to their weight program. But the smart ones who do include it come away with a more shapely pair of legs and a firm, tight rear end. Guys and gals alike, appreciate the differentiation between the two, and continue to dedicate their efforts into the further development of that particular area.

Properly executed, lunges will further define and separate the muscles of the thigh, while greatly increasing one's leg and groin flexibility. The sooner you realize its importance, the sooner you will achieve optimum results.

THE DREADED BLEG

Women seem to find this exercise especially important in getting rid of the *BLEG* look. Bleg is a term a colleague of mine came up with when referring to the shape of one's rear end, meaning you couldn't tell by looking just where the leg ends and the buttocks begins, they just sort of blend together to form a *bleg*.

Instead, there should be a definite distinction between the two, an enhanced beauty of one's natural curves.

BODY POSITION

At first, this exercise may appear to look easy, but on the contrary, it is one that will require a little more practice, combined with a certain sense of balance and coordination.

Proper form and execution is just as important here, as it is in all of the other previous exercises. Just because I have presented it only as an option in this program, is no reason not to take it just as seriously.

BEGIN

Begin from a standing position, with a bar or broom handle securely resting behind your neck. (Use little or no weight)

STEP 1

Smoothly step forward in a lunging motion, out far enough so that your foot lands flat on the floor with the forward leg bent somewhere near a 90 degree angle, while keeping your trail leg straight. Here, the knee should be positioned *over* the foot, not out beyond the toes.

Keep the head up, shoulders square, and the back arched.

STEP 2

Once again, smoothly, yet powerfully, push backward with the forward leg, propelling you back up to starting position. Repeat this procedure on the other leg, and continue to alternate between legs until you finish the set. Do as many as you can.

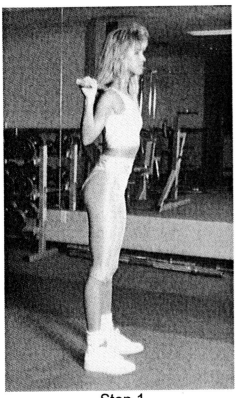

Step 1

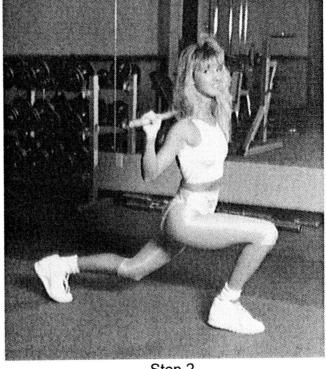

Step 2

SQUAT EXPLOSIONS

(OPTIONAL)

***************** WARNING ******************
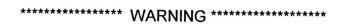

This next exercise is not for everyone and should be restricted to only those who are in excellent, all-round physical shape. You must be both flexible, and have a higher than average cardiovascular and endurance level. If you don't, I ask that you re-evaluate yourself and the practicality of executing this particular exercise and move on to the next. Remember, this is only an option, not a requirement.

****

I have included this exercise, simply because it has proven to be another one of the best all-around body exercises one can do. This includes almost every aspect of the sporting world, from professional athletes and bodybuilders, through the amateur sporting community, on down to high school athletics. Personally, there is no better way to coordinate and bind each of those individual, lower body, muscle groups worked previously, so that they can respond and perform *functionally*, as one. Think of it as an excellent way of putting on the finishing touch.

Squat Explosions will train all your lower body muscles at once. This greatly increases your endurance level, flexibility, coordination, plus it develops explosive strength and muscle responsiveness, thereby hitting almost any and every physical goal one might seek, however ambitious one may be.

Although it is a tough exercise and requires a certain amount of training, those who have made it part of their program notice enhanced toning and definition of the legs and lower torso, along with a much broader range of physical talent and athletic prowess.

PLYO-WHAT?

The Squat Explosion features the same benefits as in the traditional squat, only this particular form of exercise is based more on the principals of what is called, "*plyometrics*". This is, low impact movements with high impact results, making it a relatively safer exercise to that of others that are similar in intensity and movement. This particular form of exercise integrates not only the voluntary aspect of the muscular system, but also involves the involuntary processes as well (stretch reflex).

Many top coaches and athletes around the world have come to recognize the importance of including plyometric exercises as an added punch for those with more serious goals and ambitions. A must for any serious, *performance-oriented* workout program.

Plyometric exercises also seem to give one that added zip when it comes to managing the trials and tribulations of every day life. Use them as a way to release built up stress, or just to put that extra bounce in your step on your way to work.

BODY POSITION

Position yourself the same way you did as in the earlier Squat exercise, again, using zero resistance. Use a broom handle or an empty bar resting across the back of the shoulders.

BEGIN

With head up, back in locked position, and feet shoulder-width apart, the main objective is to forcefully jump as high off the floor as you possibly can, yet, land smoothly and safely each and every time.

STEP 1

Gently lower yourself to a full squatting position as far as flexibility will allow. *Assuming you are in elite condition and since no weight is being used, the full squat is accepted here.*

STEP 2

Next, begin the upward movement SLOWLY for the *first few inches*, in order to lessen the chance of injury to the knee joint.

Then EXPLODE, jumping straight up as high as you can off the floor as if you are trying to punch your head through the roof.

STEP 3

Land with knees slightly bent to help cushion the landing, thus making for a SMOOTH and gentle transition back down to full squat position again. Without resting, repeat and do as many as you can to finish out the set.

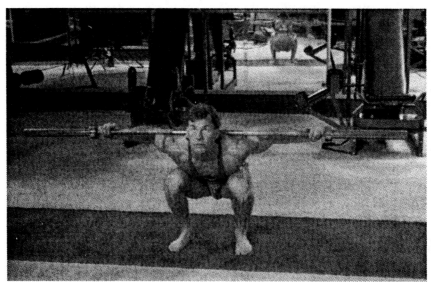

Step 1

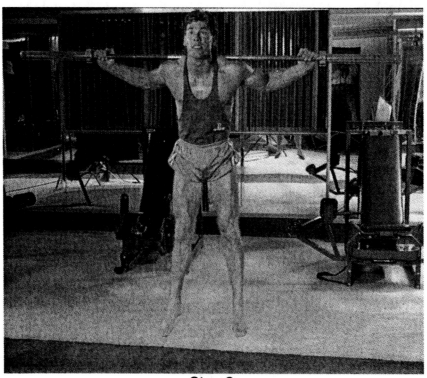

Step 2

Eventually learn to develop a rhythm that is smooth, powerful and consistent. By doing so you will find the rewards to be greater and easier to come by.

Due to the intensity and high level of cardiovascular activity involved, it is imperative that proper breathing technique is used. Inhale deeply as you lower yourself, then exhale as you explode upward.

Be aware that it is not uncommon to experience a feeling of light-headedness or dizzy spells during or immediately afterwards. It may be necessary to take a little more time to recuperate between sets.

Always use your head, combining that with caution. Eventually, you will learn through experience, how to better determine your limits.

LATERAL RAISE

(OPTIONAL)

This exercise called the Lateral Raise, will put the finishing touches on that same deltoid-shoulder region which you have just previously worked. Only this time, the emphasis will be put on the middle and rear delts. They sometimes tend to lack adequate stimulation by doing the traditional frontal press only.

Adding this exercise immediately after the Overhead Press will almost instantly amaze you in the results you will see and feel. It will be no time at all before you finally begin to notice a more defined and newly developed set of shoulder muscles. Including the Lateral Raise into your routine ensures yourself of getting that balanced, full rounded shoulder.

BODY POSITION

Assume a standing position with head up and feet in a stance that feels most comfortable to you. The arms should be fully extended except for a slight bend in the elbow to relieve possible stress on the elbow during the exercise motion.

BEGIN

Begin with the dumbbells in the lower position near the thigh area, while bending slightly forward at the waist.

STEP 1

In a relaxed manner and starting from a dead stop, raise the dumbbells in a wide circular motion out from your side, all the way up until the dumbbells are even with your shoulders.

STEP 2

Then gently lower your arms in that same wide circular motion back to starting position. Repeat until you have finished the set.

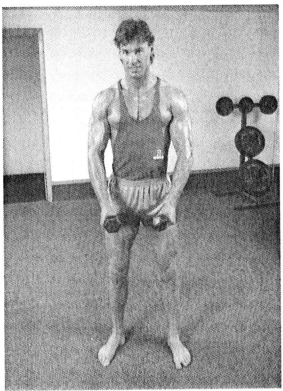

Step 1

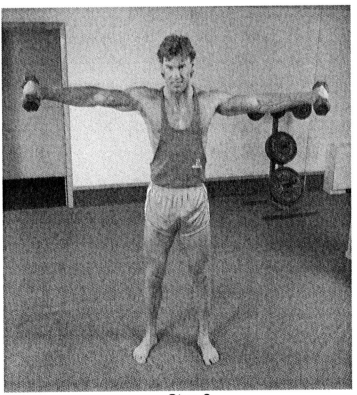

Step 2

CALF RAISE

(OPTIONAL)

The Calf Raise exercise is another option for those considered a little more picky when it comes to wanting and having the ideal leg. Often times, it is the gals more than the guys who highly value and appreciate a finer toned, enhanced calf area.

Gender aside, the addition of the Calf Raise exercise to your workout regimen will directly stimulate, strengthen, and tone those remaining muscles in the lower leg. Whereas before, although stimulated en route by more of an indirect manner, the calf and surrounding muscles were never actually targeted as they are in this form of exercise.

By comparison, the calves are the smallest muscle group in the leg and can be worked much the same as the abdominal muscles, every day. Of course, it all depends upon your goals and aspirations regarding this particular area. I leave it completely up to you. You can work them every day or simply add them to your scheduled legs-only day.

Since they are one of the smaller muscle groups, they respond best to high rep sets entered somewhere towards the end of your workout period. Shoot for at least 25-30 reps for each set.

MIXING IT UP --> (*a time saving tip*)

For those who want to try it, one can make better use of their time by using this little time-saver.

Regardless of whether you are working your upper or lower body program at the time, I personally prefer to alternate my sets of Calf Raises with my everyday Abdominal work.

> For example:
> Instead of resting idly after completing a set of Sit-Ups, I jump right in and do a good set of Calf Raises. Then, with little hesitation, I tackle another set of Sit-ups, then back to Calf Raises, Sit-ups, Calf Raises, and so on, until I've finished my program designated 3 or more sets, always with the intention of executing as many as I possibly can during each and every set.

This procedure is not as exhausting as it may sound. It enables one muscle group to adequately recover while working another, thus conveniently cutting the time factor in half, as well as capturing the added benefit of a somewhat sustained heart rate throughout.

Try it at a pace that is right for you. If not, that's fine too. This was only a suggestion.

BODY POSITION

Choose a weight that you feel you can safely handle, or simply start with an empty bar or broom handle until you gain in confidence and proper balance.

Feet should begin around shoulder-width apart with the front balls of your feet up on blocks or a 2" by 4" board.

BEGIN

Position your feet on the board as shown. Legs should remain straight so that you feel a sufficient stretch in the calves themselves.

(If balance is a problem, try switching to equally weighted dumbbells in each hand down at your side. If all else fails, place the board so that you face a wall. Using no weight, extend one or both hands out in front for balance.)

STEP 1

Rise up on your toes as high as you possibly can, making absolutely sure that it is the calves doing most of the work.

STEP 2

In a smooth and gradual manner, lower back down to starting position. Repeat this movement until you have finished the set, always with the intent of doing as many as you can.

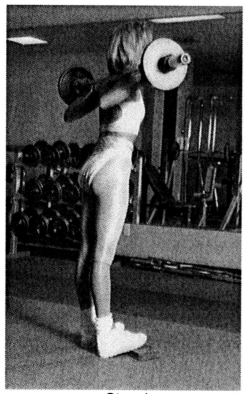

Step 1

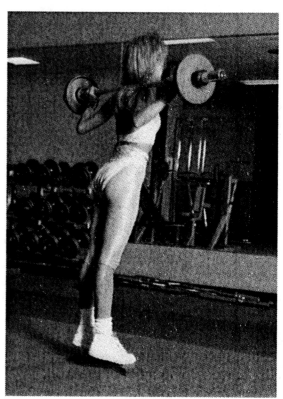

Step 2

This exercise is another that is similar in feel and effect to that of the incline curl expressed earlier, in that if done correctly, you will no doubt experience some sort of muscle burn.

This is your body's way of making a positive statement about what you've done. It simply means your doing it right (unless of course it becomes a pain of the joint or something other than routine discomfort).

SIDE TWIST

(OPTIONAL)

This particular variation of abdominal work is excellent for putting on the finishing touches towards a tighter, more toned stomach area. Side Twists not only add cuts and definition, but also greatly benefit ones flexibility throughout the upper torso. The entire range of lateral muscles that make up the side, stomach, and lower back region are directly worked, stretched, and sufficiently stimulated.

They can be included as a last minute exercise right before quitting, in turn, capturing the personal satisfaction and consciousness of achieving complete range stimulation, as well as making the transition into warm-down.

BODY POSITION
Stand upright with legs comfortably set around shoulder-width position, using a broom handle resting across your back as sort of a hanger for the arms. Lightly grasp the handle making sure to bend a little at the elbows.

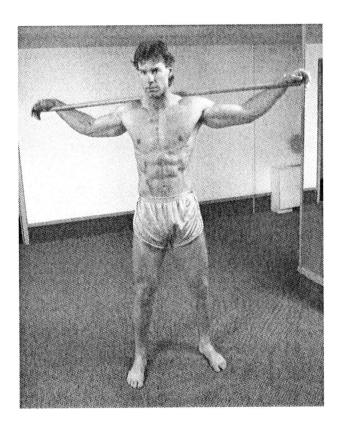

Before jumping right in, be sure to start out easy for the first few reps, or until your upper body and especially lower back, become accustomed to such twisting activity as this. The average fitness enthusiast is usually not physically prepared to go all out right at first. Most find themselves somewhat limited on just how far to the side they are actually able to twist before experiencing minor discomfort or actual pain. In short, although the movement is relatively simple, there is no reason not to begin with just as much caution here as you would in any other exercise.

STEP 1

Twist fully to one side as far as your flexibility will allow, yet, always maintaining tension on the abdominals throughout.

STEP 2

Without pausing, twist on over to the other side, in turn, developing a smooth, consistent rhythm. Repeat both steps back and forth until you have done as many as you can on each set, without excessive jerking or breaking form.

Shoot for at least 25, preferably 50 or more if possible.

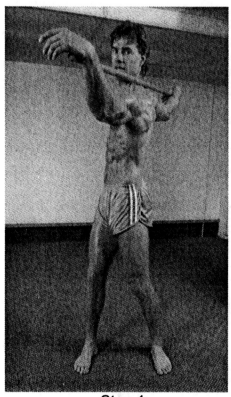

Step 1

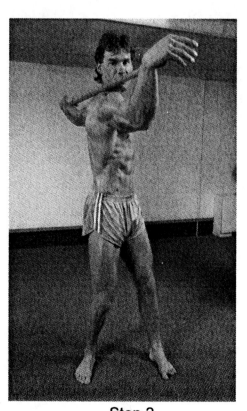

Step 2

********************* CAUTION *********************

Never swing or twist using a bar with added weight. Injury to the lower spine could occur. Always use an un-weighted bar or broom handle.

****

ORDER UP

The exercise listing given below is just that, an organized list and nothing more. If you have chosen to incorporate one or more of the specialized exercises given in this chapter **into your main program**, the order into which those should be entered should look like this.

RECOMMENDED ORDER OF EXERCISES

<u>Upper Body workout</u>   <u>Lower Body workout</u>

Upper Body workout	Lower Body workout
WARM-UP	WARM-UP
a) BENCH PRESS	a) SQUAT
b) HORIZONTAL DUMBBELL FLYE	b) LEG EXTENSION
c) OVERHEAD PRESS	c) LEG CURL
d) **LAT RAISE**	d) **LUNGES**
e) TRICEP EXTENSION	e) **FULL SQUAT EXPLOSION**
f) BENT-OVER ROWING	f) **CALF RAISES**
g) INCLINE CURL	g) BENT-KNEE SIT-UP
h) BENT-KNEE SIT-UP	h) AB-CROSS BURNOUT
i) AB-CROSS BURNOUT	i) SIDE TWIST
j) **CALF RAISE**	WARM-DOWN
k) **SIDE TWIST**	
WARM-DOWN	

This is not in any way meant to suggest that you must do each and every exercise that is given, this is merely to be used as a standard order of placement.

EXERCISE ADDITIONS

As you may already know, there are many other exercises that were not included in the previous weight training program. Many of which you have probably read about or observed others doing. But as I have stated earlier in the introduction of this book, I have purposefully selected <u>only</u> those particular exercises that will yield the faster, more productive returns, in relation to the amount of time and effort spent.

Most of us do not have that extra one or two hours or more each day it would take to get all of the additional variations of weight training in. Nor do we have the want, or quite possibly the need. Unless you are a full time athlete or professional bodybuilder, it's fairly safe to say that most of us just cannot fit that much into our day-to-day lifestyle, and yet maintain a full time job, plus quality time for the family, friends, and so on.

Granted, with the ever-growing bombardment of eye-catching TV ads along with certain hard core fitness magazines, each displaying physiques of massive muscled perfection, it's little wonder many feel *overly motivated* to try and reach out for more and more. Such influences as this progressively lead some to feel the urge to add more and more exercises in order to achieve the same results. A spell that is sometimes hard to break.

Although these kinds of tools can be great incentives and something to help give you a kick in the pants once in a while, you must realize that most of those featured are professionals. They tend to approach the sport of fitness and bodybuilding as a job, some making it their only job. It is where each individual body part is worked to its' extreme, then further isolated with a series of even more diverse forms of exercise, thus requiring a much higher level of intensity, dedication and experience. But overall, for the 99.9% remainder of the American mainstream, there should be no comparison.

As far as most of us are concerned, other body parts such as the hands, forearms, neck, and so on, although not worked directly, will be sufficiently stimulated in an indirect manner by way of the exercises given in this book. In other words, it would be almost impossible for them not to be stimulated.

However, if you feel the need to go that extra step and add other exercises, *and still be able to make it all work*, great, feel free and encouraged to do so. Just be sure that what you have chosen will contribute to your efforts, not deter from them. Because feeling good about what you're doing is what it's all about, <u>but only so long as everything else is kept in perspective</u>, including you!

GOING THAT EXTRA, *EXTRA* STEP

After a period of time, long after the weeding out process between the doers and the dropouts have taken place, there always seems to be a select few that continually reach out for more.

It's a time when they have found the rewards of their efforts so stimulating they find themselves wanting to go one step further than ever planned. Steps that were in the beginning, beyond comprehension of accomplishment, a steam-rolling effect that breeds more success and more DRIVE.

So, for those high achievers out there, this last remaining exercise *concept* is for you.

PAIN BARRIER

You're no doubt familiar with concepts like the "sound barrier", "mind barrier" and so on, but what about the "*pain barrier*" and the ability to work through it in relation to exercise.

This is entirely different from the definition or type of pain as previously discussed in chapter five. This is a unique sort of feeling, much like muscle burn, one that is looked upon in a more positive light. Working through the pain barrier allows one to increase physical results dramatically, mainly through intense isolation and further tearing down of muscle tissue, (that being part of the muscle building process).

It can be described as a specific point in any one set, when you feel an intense burning in the muscle, at, or near muscle exhaustion. This sensation is due primarily from the buildup of lactic acid in the muscle tissue. It's when the blood becomes unable to carry this acid out of the muscle fast enough, before it forms again during the constant movement of exercise. It is here, when that particular muscle is screaming at your brain loud and clear, "STOP! I can't go on!"

However, if you have confidence in what you are doing and are highly in tune with the body, it is possible to go beyond this wall of pain and finish **an extra rep or two, or three, or even four,** somehow working through the body's own natural response to quit. This type of intense mental and physical training further develops the mind-body link, in turn, strengthening the control you possess over your body and its' respective physical limits.

You'll never know how far you can go until you try, for if you can conquer the mind, you can surely conquer the body. And when that happens, that stack of goals you set long ago is just a gnats whisker from being reality.

Congratulations, you're almost there!

CHAPTER ELEVEN:

WARM-DOWN

Just as in warming up, the emphasis placed on warming down should be equally the same. It is a period after a workout session when you allow your body to *gradually* slow down, often referred to as the cooling down period. This crucial time provides the body the opportunity to expel the various toxins and chemicals that were produced during exercise.

Sitting down immediately after vigorous exercise is very unhealthy and extremely hard on your body. Some have been known to experience dizzy spells, induced muscle cramping, nausea, or even faint due to the sudden cessation of strenuous exercise. By neglecting a proper warm down period after each training session, you unnecessarily increase the amount of abuse that eventually causes your body to rebel.

Given this, there are many various methods of warm down exercises in which to choose from, each dependent upon certain factors. Such factors as *the type of activity you have just finished, the intensity in which it was performed,* and *your present physical condition.* Listed below are the primary ones that seem to be most popular. Choose the one you like best or something similar in nature for an easy period of 5-10 minutes, followed by an adequate stretching routine as outlined further in this chapter.

WALKING	OUTDOOR BICYCLING
STATIONARY BIKE	SWIMMING
JOGGING	TREADMILL

WORKS FOR ME!

Weather permitting, my personal favorite is usually a brisk jog after a weight training workout. I can set whatever pace that suits my fancy to whatever feeling or mood I happen to be in, as long as I keep it enjoyable.

For me, there is no other warm down exercise that totally tunes you in to the muscles you have just worked, both physically and mentally. At times, it becomes almost spiritual, a feeling of being one with yourself and everything around you. I have always considered myself lucky to be able to do my running out in the country, usually after dark on a back road under a moonlit sky. With a good days work and another workout behind me, I come in full view of natures gifts, and marvel at all of the good Lords' creations. Bright stars, clean air, and with thoughts only to myself, I find jogging to bring me a sense of peace and contentment from within, in turn, readying me for a good nights sleep and another day of challenges and opportunities.

Hopefully, the choice you make will be as rewarding and enjoyable as mine.

STRETCHING AND FLEXIBILITY

Included as part of any warm-down period, should be a series of stretching exercises followed soon afterwards. It doesn't have to be very time consuming or intense, just not left out.

Stretching for the purpose of maintaining flexibility is strongly recommended for everyone, *especially* those who have just undergone a weight training workout. Unfortunately, many still continue to neglect or down-play the emphasis of what a good stretching routine will do towards maintaining overall health.

Also, stretching can be used as yet another helpful tool in our "Physical Results" arsenal. A tool for measuring the range of motion of a joint. This range of movement will all depend upon the condition of three distinct physical structures. They are; the elasticity of the muscles, tendons, and ligaments of that joint. Each of these structures will stretch, but only so far and so fast.

Athletes

Increasing or maintaining ones flexibility is essential for two important reasons. One is to enhance physical performance, and the second is to reduce the chance of injury.

Top athletes continue to strive to move faster, jump higher, react quicker, and reach farther, all of which require flexibility training.

Teenagers

During the teenage years, the body is growing and changing so rapidly, that it is just as imperative to remain flexible at this time, as any other age group. If you begin to make an effort now, you no doubt will learn to appreciate those earlier efforts more and more as the years go by.

Seniors

Well, someone older might say, "I'm not an athlete OR a teenager, why should I stretch?"

As the years go by, the body continually undergoes those compressional forces created by gravity. This, combined with decreasing activity levels, will play an important part toward the effect it will have upon the entire body structure, leaving no one OR *age group* exempt.

Those smart seniors who stretch faithfully will continue to enjoy a healthier spine, better posture, and an all around more active lifestyle than those who do not.

The Average Bear

Can't find a group to place yourself in? How about forming your own and calling it "the average bear" group. One that befits all others bar none.

Again, the importance of flexibility remains the same here also. In fact, *flexibility training for one and all is probably **just as** important, as the widely emphasized dynamic duo, DIET and EXERCISE.* Bluntly put, IT'S A MUST!

OK, so even if it's not your normal, prescribed time to stretch. Just remember, anytime you feel the need, IS a good time. Especially after long periods of sitting at the desk, wheel of a car, or on your feet all day at the checkout line. At one time or another, it is something your body craves.

Even before bed, a light, easy stretching session is an excellent way to relax yourself for a good nights sleep, particularly after a hard days work, compounded by tension and stress. Try it, and eventually make it one of your regular day and nighttime rituals.

STRETCHING KNOW-HOW

Before you begin, there are a few things you should know about the act of stretching.

The first, is that you should try to stretch each joint *slowly,* as far as it is able to go *comfortably.* Do not push to the point of pain. The rules of safe stretching are as follows; *slow, gentle*, and *sustained.*

Only after reaching a comfortable point during the stretch, should you then attempt to apply a small amount of pressure in an effort to extend the joint just a little bit further, but only to the point of a slight tugging.

Try to hold this position for up to 30 seconds or more while allowing time for the muscles, tendons, and ligaments the opportunity to relax and extend.

For those whose condition is questionable, begin by stretching for shorter periods of time, somewhere around 5-15 seconds each until flexibility increases. This entire procedure should be repeated two or three times for each stretching exercise that you do.

All in all, always try to put your mind at ease. Relax and breathe deeply. Do your best to eliminate any and all remaining body tension and inhibitions. Teach yourself to *feel* what's going on, not fight it.

BEGIN

As you did in the "Warm-Up" chapter, you must now choose and develop on your own, a series of stretching exercises that more closely resembles and stimulates those areas in which you have just worked. In other words, review and analyze what parts were affected, then stretch accordingly.

To give you something to go by, I have included the following examples in which to choose from, beginning with the more familiar ones, to the more specific and targeted.

Forward Bend

Begin from a standing position with feet shoulder width apart. Slowly bend over and allow the arms to hang down. Try to keep the knees straight while giving the lower back and hamstrings a chance to relax and stretch. Eventually, try to reach your toes without bouncing or straining. You should feel it in the lower back and hamstrings.

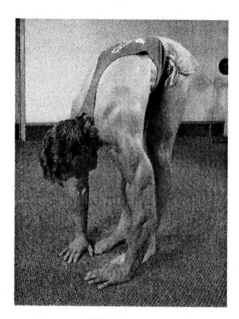

Side Bend

Stand with feet shoulder-width apart. Take one arm at a time and reach over your head as far as possible, over to the opposite side. Keep the arm over your head, disallowing it to fall too far down in front of the face. This will ensure a good stretch of the lower back and side.

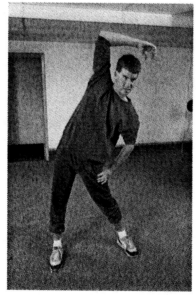

Lunge

The Lunge stretch is much the same as the Lunge exercise explained previously in the program, except you can emphasize additional areas by smoothly shifting your weight from the front to the rear. Keep the head up and the back straight.

After finishing one leg, alternate and do the other in the same manner. You should feel it in the hips, buttocks, hamstring, and all the way up the extreme upper thigh at the point where the leg connects to the torso.

If necessary, grab a chair or couch along one side to aid in balance and control.

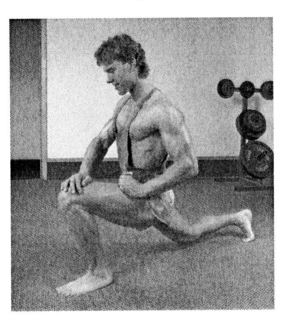

Leg Spread

Sit on the floor with the legs spread out wide as far as flexibility will allow. In a relaxed fashion, either extend your arms forward and near the floor, or grab a stationary object in front of you and carefully pull yourself down to the floor until you begin to feel a good stretch. Try to hold it for 15-30 seconds.

After several seconds have gone by, you should begin to slowly creep closer to the floor as your inner thigh and groin muscles stretch and begin to relax. When you begin to feel pain, raise up for a short time, then start again.

While in the same position, reach one arm over the top of your head as in the Side Bend stretch. Reach over to the opposite leg in the attempt to touch your opposite toe, if you can, with your head close to or touching the knee. Hold for 15-30 seconds, then switch and do the same thing on the other leg. You should feel it in the side, lower back, and hamstring.

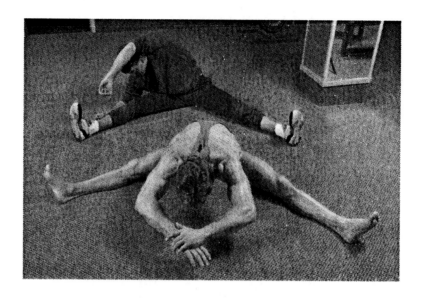

Butterfly Stretch

Assume a sitting position on the floor with both feet tucked tightly in front of your groin area. Grab the ankles and slowly bend over while applying down pressure to the legs with your elbows as shown in the picture. This is an excellent groin and inner thigh stretch.

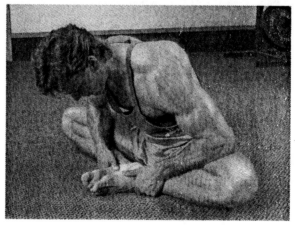

Quad Stretch

You begin in a sitting position on the floor with the arms to your side or behind you for balance. Raise the buttocks off the floor and get up on your toes. Do one leg at a time.

162

Keep one knee down and *pointing directly out to the front of you,* while at the same time leaning back with the upper body, until you feel the thigh muscle begin to stretch. Hold, then repeat the same procedure on the other leg.

Another choice for stretching the upper thigh muscles is probably familiar to most as an old standby. From a standing position, grab an ankle from one foot and pull it up behind you in a tightly tucked position. If you want more, bend over and use the other arm to touch the opposite toe.

If balance is a problem, use a chair or any other stable object with the other hand for use as a crutch.

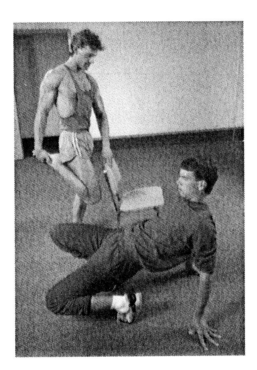

Calf Stretch

You can do this particular stretch one of two ways. The first is to position the front balls of your feet on the edge of some stairs or a thick board. Allow the heel to stretch downward while keeping the knee fairly straight. Make sure you hold onto a wall or handrail for balance.

If stairs are not available, assume a position as if you are attempting to push over a large tree. With arms outstretched and overhead, give yourself a pretty good lean into a wall, pole, or other solid object while bending one leg to the front, **but keeping the other leg straight out and behind you in a steep angled position.**

The farther back you place the straightened leg, the better the stretch in the calf, as long as the knee does not bend and the leg remains locked. Do one leg at a time.

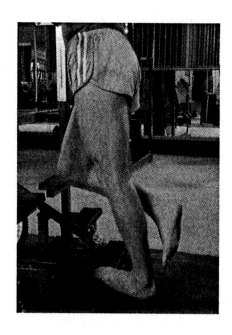

Pectoral Stretch

Stand in a doorway and place the forearms against the door frame while keeping the upper arms parallel with the floor. Step forward and lean inward with the chest. The arms should be pushed backward giving a good stretch to the chest and shoulder area.

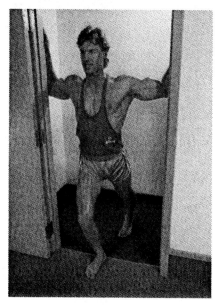

Shoulder Stretch

Begin by sitting on the floor with feet together and both hands behind your back. If possible, interlock the little fingers of both hands, (if you can't, strive to keep them as close to one another as flexibility will allow) then raise the buttocks upward as high as possible.

If you can, go one step further by shifting your center of gravity forward and to the rear, thus ensuring a full and complete stretch of the shoulder joint.

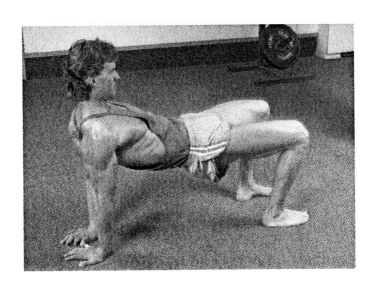

Bicep Stretch

Use a solid vertical object such as a doorway, pole or something similar. Reach straight out with one arm and hook the fingers on the edge. Slowly twist your upper body opposite the arm you are stretching. The farther you twist, the more the stretch of the bicep and shoulder. Then switch and do the other arm.

Rather than hooking the fingers on something, try pressing the thumb side of the hand against the doorway or wall with palms facing downward as shown. This method is great for further targeting of the bicep muscle.

Remember, the arm must be extended straight out to your side, not angled too far down or too high over your head.

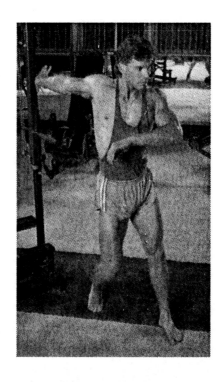

Tricep Stretch

Raise one arm at a time in a tucked position, as far behind the head as possible. Apply additional pressure with help from the other arm, by carefully pressing the elbow backward (not sideways).

If flexibility is a problem, a towel pulled downward behind the back can be used as an alternative.

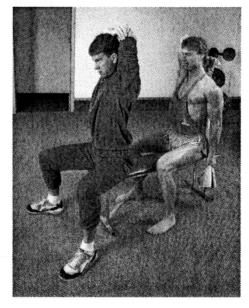

Lat Stretch

To stretch those big muscles that run down the side and make up much of the back, this stretch seems to really do the trick. Grab a solid vertical object such as a pole or doorway. Bend slightly at the knees and lean backwards using the arm for support. Shift your weight to the extreme side, whichever one that provides the best stretch. Typically, you really feel it by rotating your hips *outward,* away from your outstretched arm. If you don't get it right away, keep trying. You'll eventually get it.

Alternate and do the same on the other side.

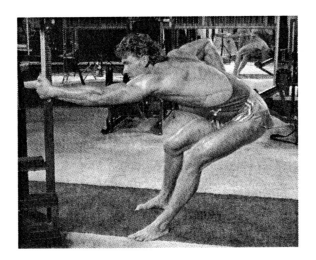

Abdominal Stretch

The abs can be stretched several different ways. The first is to assume a push up position on the floor, only in this instance, you should try and relax the abs, allowing the midsection to sag downward. Keep the head up.

Or, you can stand up straight with arms extended over the head, reaching as far behind you as possible without falling backwards.

Another favorite, is to lightly hang from a doorway or an overhead chin up bar in sort of a backward "C" fashion.

Begin by standing approximately two feet from the door opening. Reach up and lightly grasp the top and lean forward, allowing the midsection to protrude forward. In both instances, go only far enough to feel a good stretch in the abdominal region. If you force it by going too far you could end up hurting your lower back.

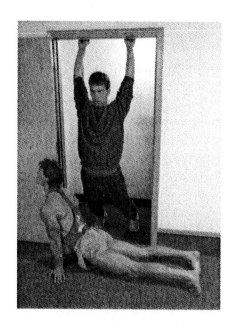

Spinal Twist

Begin by assuming a sitting position on the floor with legs together and out front. Take one foot and place it outside the knee of the other leg. Next, twist your body inward and place the opposite elbow against that knee. Apply a slight amount of pressure against the knee in an attempt to turn and look *as far behind you as possible*. This will have a direct effect upon the hip region, along with the lower spine and torso. Hold, then switch and do the other leg.

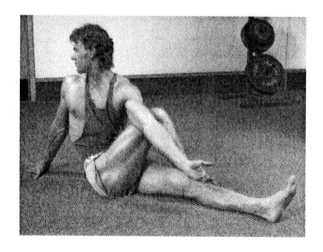

Bar Hang

The bar hang stretch is an additional incentive for maintaining a healthy spine, especially after lifting weights. It is as simple as sounds.

Lightly grasp a chin-up bar overhead in a shoulder width position to start. Do not over grip. (You can vary the width of your hand grip later, however you feel the need.) Allow yourself to hang in a semi-relaxed fashion, aiming to take the pressure off the spine.

To further enhance this feeling, slowly and carefully twist your lower body from side to side, holding it for a moment each time.

EXTRA EFFORT

Those of you who experience further flexibility problems will probably have to spend a little extra time and effort than those who don't. In other words, make it more of a priority than some of your stronger areas of your training program.

Still, there are so many more stretching techniques and practices available, I have given you only but a handful of what I consider the basic ones. If you feel the need for more of a choice, or the ones given to be too difficult, I recommend you consult your physician or local library in locating further information on specific flexibility and stretching techniques.

There are many good books and articles that specifically relate only to stretching programs and nothing else. By doing a little extra research on your part, you should be able to ensure yourself of finding that perfect stretching program tailor made for you.

CHAPTER TWELVE:

AEROBICALLY SPEAKING
(Fat Loss, Weight Control and Endurance Training)

So, are you serious about losing that extra fat? I mean really serious? How about look better, feel better? Or perhaps you merely want to increase your overall fitness and endurance level a little more?

Well here it is, and do yourself a favor, DO NOT read this chapter and then give up before even giving it a try. There is nothing more frustrating than showing someone the how-to's of physical success than to have them say, "Oh, I've tried something like that before and it just wasn't for me. Isn't there some other way?"

Come on now, be honest with yourself. Have you *really* tried? Did you make the full commitment? Is it something you've always wanted, but not THAT bad? All are questions only you can answer.

Unfortunately, in the highest percentage of cases, most fitness failures or setbacks are most often due to inadequate follow through of said instruction (going half way), or just plain laziness. In other words, one finds the degree of self-control or type of exercise required to reach their goals to be more effort than they are willing to put out.

It is here where you must STOP! You must accept, right here and right now, that the process of losing and regulating weight, or just getting in better, over-all shape is not a free ride and will require absolute effort on your part.

Likewise, just as in the adjoining weight training program, you must have that *want* and *desire* to do what it takes, and follow each method of instruction to the letter. No excuses, no buts, and no shortcuts, just do it!

I'll guarantee you, if you remain positive and apply these *most direct route* principles religiously, your goals and aspirations WILL happen. But it just doesn't stop here. The probability is high that you're way of life as you know it, could very easily turn around into a more prosperous and fulfilling environment. And I don't mean just physically.

For if you acquire the inner discipline it takes to CONTROL and SHAPE your body through diet and exercise, then there is no reason not to be able to CONTROL and SHAPE the immensity of all life's' other challenges as well.

You CAN have it all! Whether it's a whole new you, or simply an improved version, it's yours for the making. So take a deep breath and start thinking positive. Here we go!

DIET

Yup! From out of no where, the other half of the dynamic duo strikes again. Hopefully by now, you know the importance of eating healthy when it comes to any method of weight control. It should now be a matter of mere common sense.

Sadly, most people know about this primary element of fitness, but continually search for that all-encompassing magic solution. A human trait that always looks for the easiest way out in hopes of requiring little or no change on their part. I guess it all comes down to the old adage of wanting the cake, and eating it too, pardon the choice of words.

EXERCISE - DID YOU KNOW.....?

When it comes to weight control, more specifically, *fat loss,* one is either successful or unsuccessful in their attempt. In the long run, there's just no in between. In this, the strategy is simple and absolute.

There is not one, successful, weight management program out there that can be designated complete, without involving some kind of *PHYSICAL EXERCISE*.

Again, eating healthy by itself is not the answer. Although you may have your own preconceptions of what exercise is good for, you may be pleasantly surprised in the multi-dimensional role it plays in losing and regulating weight. Included in the following few paragraphs is only a brief, but essential overview of what you should already be familiar, if not, at least, NOW be aware of.

1) **Did you know**; the act of exercise itself burns little in total calories, compared to what is needed daily to lose or regulate weight?

   For example, you may go through 30 minutes of an aerobic class or tip-toed on a treadmill and burn only a few hundred calories. If your lucky, it would be enough to equal burning off one piece of pie or a peanut butter and jelly sandwich.

   Instead, you must use exercise as a way to *RETRAIN your body's own metabolic system*, so it will continue to efficiently burn calories even long after you have quit exercising, sort of like a physical re-programming.

   More than likely, back when you were a child or even in high school, you were probably unconsciously more active, thereby maintaining a higher metabolic rate. This enabled you to eat just about whatever you wanted and get away with it. Youth was also on your side.

However, as you grew older and became less active, your metabolic rate began to gradually slow down, decreasing the efficiency in which you burn your food. Although the decrease of your body's metabolism is slow and gradual, it does eventually happen, thus having a tendency for fat accumulation to creep up on you over a period of time. This often leads one to wake up one morning, casually glance in the mirror and say, "Where did that come from?"

Understand that by keeping the same eating habits you had when you were younger, **and not exercising** or staying active as you grow older, you significantly lower your metabolic rate and proceed to gain weight.

2)   **Did you know**; becoming less active also changes your *lean body mass to fat ratio*? In other words, your body tends to gain more in fat over a period of time, which in turn, offsets that fundamental balance and proportion of proper muscle/bone relationship.

Studies have shown that those who are less active and over the age of 20, **lose a half a pound of muscle every year**. Even if the weight continues to remain the same, that lost half pound of muscle will eventually be *replaced* by fat, (not turned into fat as many still believe). It may not seem like that big of a deal at the time, but look what happens;

Like V-8 engines of the body, your muscles, large or small, require fuel to sustain themselves, <u>constantly</u>. Whether playing, walking, eating, or even sleeping, they are always in need of, and continually burning calories for fuel in order to survive, 24 hours a day.

Whereas fat, primarily, requires nothing, so therefore burns nothing. It just sits there waiting to be used like some fuel storage depot, thus belonging in a class all by itself.

Consequently, the resulting effects of long-term muscle loss and what it means to you is this; those extra calories that would have been burned by lost muscle are, you guessed it, then stored as fat. So, it only stands to reason that the greater the percentage of **lean muscle buildup** than that of fat, the higher your body's metabolism and fitness level will be.

In short, *the bigger the engines and more of them, the more fuel they will burn.*

Therefore, you should strive to increase your lean body mass (bone and muscle tissue) and reduce fat content **<u>through exercise</u>**. I believe this to be a key element in the understanding process of not only ridding oneself of fat, but maintaining and keeping it off as well. Don't let your body turn to mush.

3)   **Did you know**; for most and with few exceptions, it's better to exercise *longer* rather than harder? Many of today's exercise newcomers as well as those more experienced are pleasantly surprised to find that long, moderate workouts give them a bigger (and safer) return in weight control, than those of the shorter, harder ones.

For as one engages in an activity of prolonged exercise, the initial fuel the body uses most is in the form of carbohydrates, which is not really what we're after. BUT, as *exercise continues*, fats then gradually take over as the primary fuel source, therefore placing the body in the proper fat burning state.

Still, many continue to conform to the notion "the harder you huff and puff, the better the results". However, recent studies continue to show otherwise. No doubt you've probably heard the expression, "no pain, no gain"? Well, for Mr. and Mrs. Mainstream this sounds pretty scary, as well it should be. Such a misconception is why so many start an exercise program and quit shortly thereafter, due mainly because of burnout and/or injury.

Actually, you should work to reach a pace that is somewhere between moderate, to somewhat hard. No more! Get to a level that you can carry on a conversation without becoming dizzy or gasping for breath. Ignore those individuals who are going faster or working harder than you. They are either in much better shape, or probably don't know what they are doing.

Always remember, whether you jog a mile in 15 minutes or run it in 6, know that you will burn approximately the same number of calories, making your only concern that of **time**. That's right, TIME! This should eliminate any confusion regarding miles or laps or whatever.   So, back off just a little and exercise.....*the aerobic way*.

EXERCISE THE AEROBIC WAY!

In order to train our body to burn fat and many of those unwanted calories, we must find a type of exercise that will safely raise our heart rate **for a sustained period of time** as just mentioned. There are many exercise programs out today that accomplish this, but often come across as too complicated and/or intimidating. So I will keep it simple by summing it up in one word: "aerobic".

The term "aerobic exercise" means, *with oxygen*. Quite simply, it is an activity or exercise that allows the body's metabolism **to effectively burn fat,** (with the possible exception of "cross-training" featured later on), aerobic training is THE MOST beneficial type of exercise to increasing one's overall fitness level and dropping unwanted fat weight. Other benefits include a higher energy level, an increased capacity for work, a reduction in stress, and an increased devotion to one's eating program.

"An-aerobic" exercise is just the opposite of aerobic, meaning *without oxygen*. A good example would be like most weight training programs. Although working with weights will build bigger fuel-burning engines and may use up some unwanted calories, it will however, have less of an effect in the **direct** burning of fat.

Just ask any one of literally millions who faithfully participate and they will tell you, *AEROBIC* exercise is where it's at, and all it takes........is to simply begin!

SIMPLY BEGIN!

STEP (A)

First of all, you must determine what your heart's individual training zone is, with age being the determining factor. This is the range in which you can safely maintain your heart rate throughout exercise for a sustained period of time, while having reached a level sufficient enough to promote fitness. It can be found in one of two ways.

The first, is to refer to the Training Zone chart to determine where you fit in. You should strive to maintain a heart rate at or somewhere between 65-80% of your maximum output. This is the range you need to be in to safely reach your desired results.

YOUR HEARTS' INDIVIDUAL TRAINING ZONE

	Heart Rate (in beats per minute)			
AGE	60% level	65% level	80% level	Max. Heart Rate
20	120	130...............160		200
25	117	126...............156		195
30	114	123...............152		190
35	111	120...............148		185
40	108	117...............144		180
45	105	114...............140		175
50	102	110...............136		170
55	99	107...............132		165
60	96	104...............128		160
65	93	100...............124		155
70	90	97...............120		150
(beginners)		[-------- Training Zone ------]		(not recommended)

175

******************** CAUTION ********************

It is NOT recommended that you exceed the 80% level for a long period of time. It could not only be dangerous, but tends to swing your body into sort of an anaerobic overdrive, whereby burning more glucose for fuel, than that of stored fats).

****

The second way, if you so choose, is to use this next simple calculation, always using the number 220 as the set standard for determining your top and bottom end training zones. (This method will give you the same information as in the previous chart, aside from helping you understand for yourself how the figures are reached.)

Subtract your age from 220, and then multiply by 65% (.65). For example, take someone who is 37 years old.

$$\begin{array}{r} 220 \\ -\ 37 \\ \hline 183 \\ \times\ .65 \\ \hline \end{array}$$

= 118.9   beats per minute at 65% maximum heart rate

$$\begin{array}{r} 220 \\ -\ 37 \\ \hline 183 \\ \times\ .80 \\ \hline \end{array}$$

= 146.4   beats per minute at 80% maximum heart rate

This shows that an individual 37 years old should try to reach and maintain an exercise heart rate, **somewhere on or between,** 120 and 146 beats per minute for the most part of their workout. This then would be this individuals training zone.

If you are a true beginner and find the 65% range to be too difficult at first, re-calculate by replacing the 65% figure with 60%. This will give you a little easier bottom number to start from, until your endurance level increases enough to move back up to at least the 65% range.

STEP (B)

Next, you must be able to find your individual heart rate **during** exercise and translate into beats per minute. You probably know it as taking your pulse.

Put your index and middle finger together and place lightly on the underside of the opposite wrist, directly below the thumb. Here you will find your "radial artery".

While using a stopwatch or watching the second hand on a clock, count your pulse beats for 10 seconds and multiply that number times 6. Or if you prefer to count longer, count the number of beats for 15 seconds and multiply by 4. Either way, this will give you your average heart beats per minute. (You should always begin the count ON a heartbeat.)

Others prefer to monitor their pulse much in the same manner, only choosing the area on the upper neck, directly below the back of the jaw bone. The pulse you will find at that spot is the "carotid artery".

If possible, get into the habit of monitoring and tracking your heart rate *during exercise*, instead of trying to figure it out as soon as you stop exercising. As you will learn, within 15 seconds or so after cessation of exercise, the heart rate begins to slow down rapidly, thus making it difficult to get an accurate reading.

An alternative elective would be to choose from many choice gadgets and electronic devices available on the market that make finding ones heart rate even simpler. They are commonly referred to as heart rate monitors. Although they seem to be a bit of an added luxury, there are those who wouldn't exercise without them.

At a glance, and without fumbling for a pulse or doing arithmetic in your head, heart rate monitors will provide you with an instant and continuous digital read out of your present heart rate throughout. They come in many forms, features, and price ranges. From a simple fingertip monitor, all the way up to the ones with specially designed, built-in computers, each depending upon individual goals and tastes. For more detailed information on heart rate monitors, I recommend you seek out a reputable sporting goods dealer.

STEP (C)

Now you must choose what aerobic exercise best suits you and your present fitness level. Listed next are the primary exercises used most to raise and sustain the heart rate.

As you read through and study each one, notice all seem to carry the same common denominator, in that each aerobic exercise directly involves the large, lower torso muscles of your buttocks and legs. Just about any time these areas are targeted during exercise, you will no doubt experience some kind of beneficial cardiovascular work.

WALKING

A very basic exercise that works well for those who should start at a very low intensity level. When results become hard to find and your heart rate is not where it should be, only then should you increase your walking pace.

You should also be aware that, with few exceptions, walking as an exercise by itself will probably not work for the average weight loss enthusiast. It will take more effort than that.

POWER WALKING

Power Walking is a step up from your average walk, combining low impact exercise with a more aggressive body style (walking at a much faster pace with an emphasis on increased arm action). It has become popular for those in poor to moderate physical condition.

JOGGING

If you find little gained by walking, maybe you should try jogging. Always start out cautiously, gradually working up to a comfortable pace in which your heart reaches its exercise training zone. Be aware that this type of exercise is more weight bearing in effect, and could result in discomfort of the joints if you push yourself too quickly, so take it easy.

After awhile, you may want to add a little variety to your jogging trail. Providing you are up to it, try tackling a hill or two, adding a few short sprints now and then, perhaps do a little cross country training through some fields or woods. Constantly challenge yourself to keep it interesting.

STATIONARY BICYCLE

This particular exercise not only proves to be an adequate aerobic fat burner, but carries with it the benefit of being non-weight bearing, unlike walking or jogging. And by choosing a slightly more specialized apparatus that adds arm and upper body action in conjunction with normal pedaling, you can assure yourself of an even better, overall conditioning effect that can make this exercise hard to beat.

Also, the stationary bike can be done indoors at a your favorite fitness facility, or in your own home, without regard to outside weather conditions. With the stationary bicycle, you have the option to ride while watching television or reading a magazine as the time ticks on by.

(Make sure the seat is adjusted properly. With the pedal at it's lowest point, your leg should be almost, but not completely straight.)

RECUMBENT BICYCLE

The recumbent bike carries the same benefits and advantages as the stationary bicycle except for the position in which you ride. Actually, you sit in what looks like an ordinary chair only that the pedals are positioned out in front, rather than below as in the more familiar style. Some say it is more comfortable to ride and provides a different feel during exercise. Regardless, it all comes down to a matter of preference.

BICYCLING / MOUNTAIN BIKING

Bicycling has become more than just a fun past time. It is not only a great exercise, but has now come into its own as a major sporting event. Those who participate in cycling, whether for sport or fun, find it to be a most effective aerobic exercise. The benefits are much the same as the stationary bike, but less monotonous and more scenic in nature.

AEROBIC CLASSES

Whether or not you are into the club scene or prefer to workout at home, aerobic-type classes or programs can be another great exercise in training your body to lose and better control weight.

Aerobic classes are provided by most health clubs and various other related organizations. They are offered under a variety of intensity levels, all from the simplest of movements, advancing up through world-class fitness levels. They also provide an often-times, much needed, class atmosphere. A chance to make new friends and relationships while preventing boredom.

However, those who prefer to do their workout at home may need further help and encouragement. That is why some prefer to choose from a long list of helpful aerobic workout videos currently available on the market. It doesn't matter what you choose, just as long as whatever it is, WORKS!

SWIMMING

Swimming is arguably labeled to be the best overall exercise that you can do. It features aerobic training by way of total body stimulation, highly targeting both lungs and muscles at the same time. Swimming also increases flexibility and full range motion of the joints. Unlike other exercises, swimming provides smooth, constant resistance, and is non-weight bearing, thus greatly reducing the chance of injury. It is also frequently used for endurance training of athletes. For those who swim, most find lap swimming to provide the best results, however, treading water is also good.

Not only is swimming prime exercise, but it's used extensively for rehabilitative therapy, treating anything from serious back and joint injuries, to stress reduction.

However, there are usually two major drawbacks that confront would-be swimmers. The first is that swimming in itself is not the best at ridding oneself of fat weight. And the second seems to be the lack of availability of a swimming pool.

For those involved, simply incorporate another aerobic exercise in with your normal swimming regimen and begin your pool search by checking with your local YMCA or internet browser.

CROSS-COUNTRY SKIING APPARATUS

In most cases, this full-body workout tends to give you more bang for your effort in relation to some of the other more popular choices, making the cross-country trainers an excellent alternative to consider. It features a non-impact alternative to weight-bearing exercises like walking and jogging, yet carries a much greater overall toning effect for the rest of the body rather than primarily working the lower half.

OTHER MACHINES

There are many other machines and choice gadgets on the market designed to raise your heart rate through exercise, most do what they advertise. Some examples include;

Treadmill
Stair Climbers
Climbing and Rowing machines
In-line Skating

You name it, it's out there. Again, you must closely evaluate your personal goals and present fitness level in order to determine which is best for you. Always play it smart. It doesn't make sense to go out and purchase a rowing machine when you have a bad back.

CIRCUIT TRAINING

Do you get bored aerobi-cising? Do as others have done by combating boredom and dull routines by the method of "circuit" training. This is where you exercise on more than one machine or apparatus during any one workout session, mixing and matching each according to your preferential moods. (Of course this usually requires a fully equipped gym.)

An example could be when one starts out on a stationary bicycle for a few minutes of warm-up, then moves over to the treadmill for several more, then on to a stair climber, rowing machine, and so forth, until your 20, 30, or 40 minute session is up, **so long as the heart rate remains in its respective training zone throughout**. You could also throw in a few weight training exercises for better balance and conditioning. Give it a try.

******************** Helpful Hint ********************

If you are still undecided on which aerobic exercise to choose, I find the indoor-tools of exercise still to be the best alternative for the masses of mainstream. Whether you have access to one of these at your favorite health club, or conveniently own something of your own at home, cardiovascular indoor tools such as the ones presented here in this chapter still seem to remain the most practical. Oftentimes boring, but practical.

Generally, it's because there happens be such a wide array of choices in which to choose, while not overly expensive to own, and yet can readily fit into just about anyone's lifestyle or busy schedule. One need not worry about weather conditions or upon the dependency on others. It is totally up to you, leaving no room for excuses. So, unless you have chosen one of the alternate routes given, DO IT INDOORS!

****

"CROSS-TRAINING" The Most Direct Route!

OK, so up to this point you've followed everything to the letter never skipping a beat but still can't seem to get over that proverbial hump. You know, the one that always seems to ride up and over your belt, or the one that puts the limit on how far that new dinner blouse will stretch. Sure, in the early stages of exercise some noticeable progress may have been made, but you still remain far short of fulfilling your true desires and aspirations. Like so many others, you feel frustrated and somewhat stalled out. What now?

Enter; *Cross-training!* (Not to be confused with "circuit-training".) If you want it bad enough and provided you're already in good shape, this is it! Above all others, Cross-training could very well be the final solution for the true goal seeking, thigh trimming, tummy tucking souls, whose only wish is to somehow, some way, break new ground toward meeting their personal goals.

What's that, you still can't find enough time for exercise? Well hang on. This is an exercise that for the most part, can effectively be done within a diminished time frame over that of standard aerobics (somewhere around 15 exercising minutes per workout). Far less than what is usually required in traditional aerobic-type exercises. So why wasn't this mentioned right from the very beginning?

Truthfully, I really wanted to. But due to the average shelf-life of all those who exercise, I felt that one must first acquire some semblance of true aerobic experience and conditioning, along with a better than average sense of body awareness and its' limitations first. In one word, *experience!*

After all, the intensity level of "cross-training" is a good step or two above standard aerobic exercise. At times, just down right intense! So, in order to stand the best chance for prolonged success, one must first be physically and emotionally p..r..e..p..a..r..e..d.

Again, nothing has changed here from any other part of this book. I still want you to take things slowly, safely, and one step at a time. I WANT YOU TO SUCCEED! Today, tomorrow, next year, 50 years from now. I want you healthy, happy, and prosperous from now on through forever. That's why!

Simply put, "Cross-training" is the concept of blending short, an-aerobic bursts of accelerated activity into traditional aerobic exercise patterns. Crossing from aerobic, to an-aerobic, back into aerobic again. It's when you attempt to elevate your heart rate up to near maximum (85%) *for short periods of time* on an intermittent basis throughout your normal aerobic workout.

For example;

- If walking is your thing, try aggressively stepping up the pace for short distances in an attempt to momentarily increase your heart rate above your normal optimum training range. (Breathing harder is part of it!) Once there, slow back down to normal pace until your heart rate drops back down into the optimum aerobic training range. Repeat this over and over throughout your normal workout.

- Joggers should try sprinting at different times. Pick those knees up, pump those arms. Shoot for 100 feet, half a block, tackle a hill or two, whatever you think it will take to get the heart rate up to near maximum for a short period of time. Then back down into a jog. Again, bringing the heart rate with it, down into the previous training range of your normal jog (not a walk). Repeat several times throughout your normal run.

- Bikers (indoors or out), rowers, you on the treadmill, you should think about accelerating at different times and/or distances, then back down to usual cruising speed. Accelerate, cruise, accelerate, cruise, I think you get the picture.

All in all, whatever type of aerobic exercise or tool you choose, consider giving "cross-training" a try! Mix it up. Challenge yourself. Do your best to keep aerobic exercise as productive and stimulating as possible. Not only will you experience energetic health and happiness, but you will soon be able to find your belt again or happily have to go shopping for that one, new, smaller blouse.

STEP (D)

In this last step, you have probably heard that the best results from standard aerobic exercise come from *no less* than 20 minutes of sustained activity, a minimum of three days per week. Realistically, for those trying to lose **fat weight**, you need to work up to 45 minutes or more (except for "cross-trainers"), 5 days a week.

But everyone has to start somewhere and that somewhere is right here and right now. If you are in doubt as to your physical shape or capabilities on where to start, use the gradual method of succession below, using the stationary bicycle as the primary example.

1st week:	ride for **2** minutes rest for **2** minutes <u>ride for **2** minutes</u> **6** minutes total	**2nd week:**	ride for **3** minutes rest for **2** minutes <u>ride for **3** minutes</u> **8** minutes total
3rd week:	ride for **4** minutes rest for **2** minutes <u>ride for **4** minutes</u> **10** minutes total	**4th week:**	ride for **5** minutes rest for **2** minutes <u>ride for **5** minutes</u> **12** minutes total

5th and 6th week: ride continuously for **10** minutes

7th and 8th week: ride continuously for **15** minutes

9th and 10th week: ride continuously for **20** minutes

And so on up to 30 minutes or more, depending on your individual goals and intensity level.

Remember, you need *at least* 20 minutes per workout, at least three days per week. Set yourself a set day and time for each workout session. An example would be like a Monday-Wednesday- Friday program.

In addition, unlike certain weight resistance exercises, an aerobic program can be done everyday if you so choose. In fact, an **everyday**, 30 minute or more aerobic routine is greatly encouraged, providing faster results for the more impatient, or simply those with higher aspirations.

If time becomes a limiting factor, break it up into smaller versions at some time throughout the day. Ten minutes in the morning before work, ten minutes during midmorning or afternoon break, ten minutes after work, whatever, whenever, and however you can. Just as long as it all adds up to 20 or more minutes total.

*************** A Note of Caution ***************

Always allow at least 5 minutes of gradual warm-up time before attempting to first reach your heart's optimum training zone. Likewise, you should allow another 5 minutes of cool down period afterwards. Refer to the exercise chart below, again using a person 37 years old as an example.

****

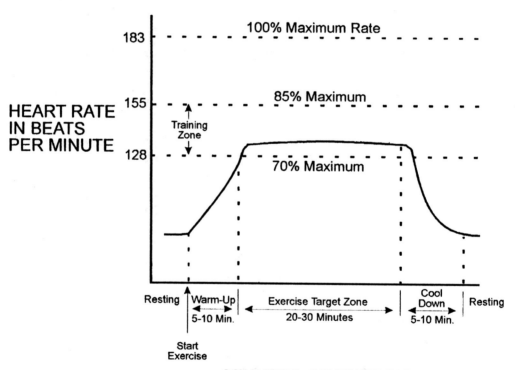

EXERCISE HEART RATE PATTERN

MINUTES OF EXERCISE

***************** Reality Check *****************

Federal guidelines now suggest 150 minutes of moderate exercise per week is what it will take for those trying to lose fat weight. That figures out to about 50 minutes/day on a 3 day/week program, roughly 40 minutes/day on a 4 day/week program and 30 minutes/day on a 5 day/week program. Preferably, a blend of aerobics, weight training, and sports.

Again, this is something you must gradually build up to. More than twenty minutes of continuous exercise could be more than you are able to handle early on. Therefore, each increase in workout time should be attacked one chunk at a time. Your success depends on it.

****

TAKE HEART AND CONQUER

At this point, each prospective workout enthusiast should take heart in knowing that for many, the hardest part of aerobic exercise is usually the first few minutes when just beginning, especially if you are one who continues to make a habit out of continually watching the clock.

It seems that during the first part of any given workout period, 20, 30, 40 minutes, whatever time frame you're into, your mind is always there nagging at you, painfully pressing home the fact that you still have what seems like a long, long way to go. This relentless body versus brain tug-of-war, all too often negatively progresses into an overwhelming, discouraging force that makes your efforts, as well as the odds of finishing, even more difficult. Those of us who routinely undertake aerobic exercise know this feeling all too well. But take heart!

Usually, it's not until you finally pass the *halfway point* in your program when you should begin to feel as though you are in more of a "cruising mode", a reassured feeling of being on the downhill side of finishing. Somehow, at this point, it doesn't appear to be quite as difficult as it once was only minutes before. In doing so, that light at the end of the tunnel seemingly gets a whole lot brighter. "That wasn't so bad, I CAN finish this after all!"

Reaching the *half way* point, THAT'S the key. That's usually when the mind begins to focus more on finishing what it started, rather than throwing in the towel.

Some even find within themselves a renewed sense of vigor and graduate to stepping up the pace little by little, day by day. Others are surprised to find themselves urged to press on even further and end up going considerably longer than first planned. For many, it becomes self-perpetuating. As confidence builds, goals expand and success becomes reality.

Here is exactly why it is so important for each of us to take heart and conquer! Rather than quit the first time things get a little on the tough side, we must instead, all learn to fight through **our own natural response of wanting to quit too soon,** by ceaselessly training and conditioning the mind and all conscience thoughts. Control your actions. Control your emotions. Control your destiny.

<u>Mind Control</u> during exercise, work on it! Because if you quit too early in the race, you will never make it to the finish line.

ENTER-TRAIN YOURSELF

This now brings up a dilemma of which no one is immune. *Boredom*, aerobic exercise's #1 adversary responsible for most failures and inconsistencies. With the possible exception of aerobic classes, climbing on a stationary bike, treadmill, or just about any other indoor aerobic activity for a monotonous 20-60 minute stretch of time while listening to your body complain is not only difficult, but often times failure-ridden.

The key here is to *keep the mind occupied and ENTERTAINED*, (this is quite unlike weight training where full and complete concentration is a must). Because no matter what the motivation factor happens to be, the majority of us who undertake aerobic exercise still require some sort of outside stimuli to keep us going. Not only for today's workout, but for those many, many more down the road.

X-out boredom by taking advantage of such things as the radio, television, magazines, or a good book, while working your way to a better you. Popping in a good movie on the VCR or listening to a home-made tape of all your favorite songs can be a real enlightenment for those who feel burdened with aerobic exercise. Quite simply, do what you have to do in order to make it as fun and comfortable as possible.

By learning to incorporate these and other helpful "entertraining-type" tools into your aerobic exercise regime, you will gladly find the mind temporarily occupied to a point, where the time literally flies by and your done before you know it. Try it, and you'll be on your way.

LOOSING THE RIGHT STUFF

Finally, for those bound and determined in making a final stand in the weight loss game, I want to leave you with something to think about that could make all the difference. The difference between getting where you want and feeling good about yourself in the process OR, failing in your quest and feeling worse than before, *again*!

DON'T be one of those obsessed with <u>continually</u> weighing yourself.

Be more realistic in your approach to self-fulfillment. True, *measurable* weight loss plays a big incentive towards staying in the fitness game. Unfortunately, many still measure the success of our diet and exercise programs entirely upon the results of what our bathroom scales show us. Resist!

In truth, scales can be most deceiving because they measure only in pounds. They have the inability to distinguish between fat loss, water loss, or the loss of lean body mass. This leads many to be overly concerned on *total* weight loss, rather than emphasizing *what exactly* has been lost.

In short, just know that there is a distinct difference in the *kind* of weight you ultimately want to lose, usually in the form of fat. Fat loss is something you cannot always ascertain by continually weighing yourself. So, pay less attention to your scales and more to what is reflecting in your *mirror*, it won't lie. Get the picture?

The Bottom Line

STEP A: Find your heart's individual training zone.
STEP B: Know how to find and determine your heart rate during exercise.
STEP C: Choose an aerobic exercise that best fits you.
STEP D: Exercise a minimum of 150 minutes per week.
STEP E: If all else fails, "Cross-train"! It's harder work, but quite effective.

SUMMARY

- Have a complete physical before starting this or any other aerobic exercise program.

- You must understand that aerobic activity isn't just the burning of a few calories through exercise, but rather more of *training* your body to increase its own metabolic furnace.

- Aerobic exercise is not as effective unless used in conjunction with a good diet plan. (There is that "D" word again.)

- Stay hydrated. Always keep that water bottle close at hand!

- Begin cautiously and gradually when starting any kind of aerobic exercise. If you begin to feel faint, dizzy, or experience unusual shortness of breath, stop immediately and consult your physician.

- Those who have more difficulty in shedding fat or reaching their target weight, should gradually increase their aerobic exercise time to 30 - 50 minutes per session, 5 - 6 days per week. (For most of us, this is closer to what it's actually going to take. I'm sorry, but this is r..e..a..l..i..t..y!)

- Remember, no matter what your present frame of mind is during any one particular exercise session, you must strive to at least reach the half-way point of your program. If you do, I can almost promise you, the last half, on through to completion, will not be as bad as the first. Can you say success? I knew you could.

- AEROBICS ALONE **WILL NOT** GIVE YOU THE COMPLETE BODY YOU WANT. Results will be even more gratifying and *long lasting* by incorporating weight training exercises as well.

  I say again, never EVER underestimate the power of weight training! Remember, larger, healthier muscles mean more calories burned, <u>constantly</u>.

- Believe it or not, refusing to properly diet and exercise will not turn your muscles into fat, rather, the unused muscles merely shrink away. However, such muscle loss, or absence of normal healthy muscle volume will be, you guessed it, <u>replaced</u> by fat.

- Walking your way to fitness is a good start, but for most, and with few exceptions, it won't be enough to reach realistic fat loss goals.

- Many times exercise programs fail, not because one does not try, but because one tries too hard, *too soon*.

- This aerobic program is NOT intended to be used only as a way to rid yourself of fat and obesity, **and then stopped**. It is an activity that should be accepted and understood as a lifetime commitment.

- For those who have chosen an aerobic-type apparatus such as a stationary bike, treadmill, or something similar in nature that come with those handy-dandy, little timer/countdown gadgets try this;

  Warm up, set your timer, then don't look at it! Don't even peek until you've completely finished and time has run out.

  Throw a towel or magazine over the digital time display, anything that will keep you from being able to constantly monitor the time. Keep the mind entertained! The time usually passes much quicker *and easier* if you do. Give it a try!

- Remember, this is NOT a *weight* loss program. It is a **_fat_** loss program! Know the difference!

- You MUST NOT neglect or skip over any of the steps A,B,C, or D. Each must be followed and carried through with equal effort and attention to detail.

No one but YOU can better your physical condition. The ball is now in your court, what are you going to do with it? Dribble down the court toward success, or pass it off and go sit with the rest of the plump and portly crowd?

CHAPTER THIRTEEN:

FOR ALL AGES
(Seniors, Teens, and Pre-teens)

What are your feelings on EXERCISE? Do you fear it? Are you intimidated by it? If you are, is it because of your age, your present health, physical problems? Perhaps you consider it too soon or too late to begin? Or is it something more? Whatever answers come to mind, there is one that should surely stick; DO IT!

I am referring to those groups on opposite ends of the spectrum that are all too often left out of the big picture. Groups important in their own right, yet often crowded out by the masses of mainstream. Those special groups being Seniors, Teens and Pre-teens. They too, have their place of function in society and must also be concerned with their health.

Unfortunately, the vast majority still continue to hold the ill-conceived notion that exercising over or under a certain age can be either hazardous, not worth the time spent, or at the very least, somewhat intimidating.

It is here where one and all must begin anew, by way of a careful, systematic attack and conquer of those fears and weaknesses that remain in all of us. Each particular individual will have to dig deep inside themselves and pull out that *want* and *desire* in order to fulfill any of their physical ambitions. Assuming you are reading this now, proves you have already taken the first step towards your success. Keep it going!

SENIORS

We will begin first with that special group of individuals that make up the elderly group, although it will not necessarily be confined to only those higher up in years. If you are sixty-five but feel more like thirty-five, you may not feel that you fit in the category of the elderly. But on the other hand, if you are thirty-five and feel more like your body is sixty-five, then you should have cause for concern and group yourself accordingly.

Remember, you feel only as old as you allow yourself to feel. If you want to keep active, you must be active, energy will create energy. In this case, the muscles of the body are no different, you either use them or lose them.

Think about it. What happens to a broken arm or leg when the cast is finally removed? Is the condition the same as when it went in? Probably not. Obviously, the *unused* muscles shrink from lack of use. Now, what happens if you treat your entire body in similar fashion? That's right! The deterioration process does not discriminate, thus bringing home the importance of staying active at any age.

With this in mind, now is as good a time as any to start thinking in a *positive* way toward exercise, regardless of your thoughts on it up to this point. It is not something to be dreaded or somehow bumped out of the way whenever you feel like it, but rather permanently accepted as a way of life, or perhaps better put, **for the rest of your life**.

First, examine for yourself what it means for the non-active or an elderly person to exercise. Then, quiz yourself and draw your own conclusions.

1) Being *independent* plays a large role for folks up in their years. With a healthy body, you will have the freedom of doing most anything you want at any time, enabling you to take care of yourself and enjoy what life has to offer. You will feel good as well as look good, needing little or no help from anyone.

2) What is old age? Is it being a senior citizen, allowing your life to be limited by disabilities, watching television in your easy chair as the clock ticks by? Using your age or disability as excuses not to become more active is a large waste. Now is not the time to let the world go by, allowing your mind and body to become weak and silent. Old age is only what you perceive it to be, or **what you allow it to become**. Old age is living the life you deserve, full of energy and vitality, resulting in harmony and joyfulness. You've worked hard all of your life to get where you are, why not get the most out of it and reap what you now deserve?

3) Today's science has without a doubt, proven that healthy, older, individuals can greatly improve their functional capacities through physical conditioning. Percentage-wise, the rate of their improvement is *almost the same as those much younger.*

4) "The importance of exercise for the elderly as listed below, comes from the Office of Aging, U.S. Department of Health and Human Services.

   • The degree of disability for seniors can be lessened through exercise.
   • Exercise helps strengthen bone mass which is weakened in the later years by osteoporosis.
   • Exercise can increase muscular strength and endurance which deteriorates through inactivity.
   • Exercise improves a person's joint flexibility and range of motion by keeping them loose and mobile.
   • Exercise improves the body's sense of balance. (Potentially reducing chances of falling.)
   • Respiratory ability and efficiency (which may gradually decrease with age). can be improved with exercise.

- Arthritis cannot yet be eliminated, but some of the painful symptoms can be relieved and flexibility increased.
- Improved circulation and a reduction in high blood pressure can be accomplished with exercise and diet.
- Mental status can be improved, plus anxiety, the blues, or mild depression can be relieved through exercise.
- The amount of oxygen (through improved circulation) can increase and enhance mental alertness."

5) *Exercise not only adds years to your life, but adds life to your years!*

ARTHRITIC PATIENTS

I feel there is a need to say something for those people cursed with arthritis. Although there is presently no cure, one must not give up.

Arthritis is a disease of the joints, which is commonly dependent upon medication for relieving discomfort. In this case, **arthritic joints should never be pushed**, just stimulated, through gentle and easy movements of exercise. With caution, body sculpting exercises like the ones in this book are most beneficial in working the joint through it's full range of motion, while improving flexibility and strengthening the surrounding muscles. This type of activity squeezes essential nourishing fluids into the joint capsule and along the entire joint surface.

The stimulation you receive from just such exercise helps keep you from *fusing up.* Remember, a little exercise for arthritic patients is better than not doing anything at all.

SENIORS, START YOUR ENGINES!

All right guys and gals, lets get started! (I prefer to use the younger implication of guys and gals, rather than ladies and gentlemen. I consider anyone in the senior group who eagerly undertakes any type of formal exercise program, still to be young at heart, and carries with them that younger, active personality, just waiting to burst out and be recognized.)

For those of you who have either been predominantly inactive, have a certain disability, or have lost most of your flexibility and endurance, I will again stress the importance of checking with your personal physician before undertaking this or any other exercise program. It is especially important for this particular age group to know where they stand physically before starting.

You should also know by now that no one is exactly the same when it comes to individual capacity for exercise. So avoid trying to stay up with your neighbor or friend by attempting to do the same workouts or routines. Never be ashamed to fit yourself into an easier exercise group. YOU alone, (with help from your physician), must be able to honestly determine what activity level best suits you and your life style. Whether your goal is to be able to walk down to the mall, or involve yourself in more social activities such as dancing, jogging, or tennis, set your goals then proceed accordingly.

Furthermore, please do not get carried away with enthusiasm. It's very easy to do, especially in the beginning. You may find that overdoing one day of exercise, may land you three days or more in bed, therefore accomplishing little, plus the added discomfort and inconvenience.

As I stated in the chapter called "Use Your Head", always listen to your body and its signals. Use the common sense the good Lord gave you. If you start to feel pain or dizziness, it's your body's way of letting you know you are beginning to overdo it. Always tune yourself in to what is going on. Finding your *exercise capacity* will take patience and care. Start out slow and easy. DO NOT OVERDO IT!

Listed next, are some basic exercises that are directed toward the senior group, focusing our primary objective towards total body stimulation through easy, low impact exercise. Since everyone will require different capacities for exercise, there will be no set standard to follow.

Simply choose and make up your own schedule from the given order of exercises, or preferably, start with the first one and follow as instructed. They begin with easy, low intensity movements (stage 1), graduating on up through the more difficult levels (stages 2 & 3).

All right, here we go!

STAGE I CONDITION

1. *Head Rotations* -> Gently move your head side to side, then forward and back. Yet, try to avoid doing this in a quick or jerky motion. Always allow your neck area to properly loosen and warm up slowly.

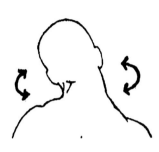 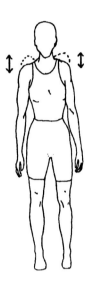

2. *Shoulder Shrug* -> Shrug your shoulders a few times while keeping arms down to your side.

3. *Trunk Twists* -> Place your hands on your hips, and twist from side to side.

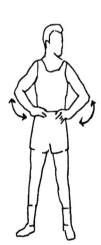 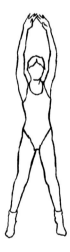

4. *Overhead Arm-Raise ->* While taking deep breaths, raise your arms above your head, then lower down to your sides, inhaling as you raise them, and exhale as they are lowered.

5. *Side Arm-Flap ->* Try flapping like a bird (slowly and smoothly) by gently moving your arms up and down.

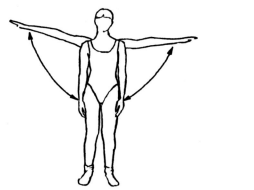 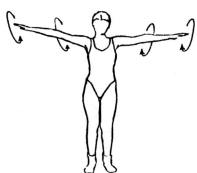

6. *Arm and Wrist Circles ->* Extend your arms out to the side while rotating them in small circles, both clockwise and counter clockwise.

   Next, maintain the extended arms, this time rotating at the wrists. Then finish with opening and closing of the hands.

7. *Seated Bend-Over ->* aids in the stretching and warming up of the back.

   Sit in a chair with legs together. Slowly lower yourself forward into your lap while allowing your arms to hang to your sides. Try to reach the position of laying your chest on top of your thighs. Relax and feel the stretch in your back. Hold for 15-20 seconds, then sit up straight. Repeat several times.

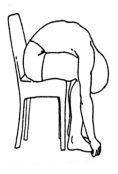 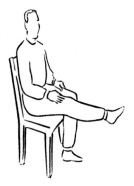

8. *Seated Leg Extension* -> will stimulate the muscles in front of your legs (quadriceps).

Begin seated in a chair with correct sitting posture and feet together. Smoothly extend one leg at a time straight out in front and lightly flex. Lower back to starting position and then repeat by alternating the other leg.

9. *Stand/Sit* -> exercise is exactly what the name implies. It will stimulate your leg and buttock muscles.

Start by sitting in a chair with proper posture, then stand up fully, again with proper posture. Sit down, and repeat.

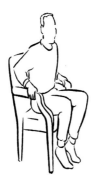 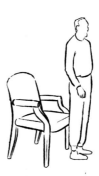

10. *Standing Knee Lift* -> is another accomplished exercise that works the leg and abdominal muscles. It also provides an increased sense of balance.

To begin, you can use the back of a chair as a crutch to aid you in balance until you can perform the exercise without it.

Stand up straight beside the back of the chair. Lift one knee as high as possible on one count and finish the second count by lowering it back again to the floor. Repeat by alternating with each leg.

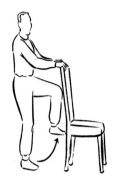 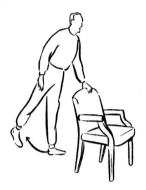

11. *Rear Leg Raise* -> will affect the lower leg, buttocks area. You will also feel a little stimulation from your lower back also.

Start by again using the back of the chair, holding on with both hands this time. Maintain a straight body line but with a slight inward lean. This will allow you to reach the chair back without bending too much at the hips or the elbows.
Smoothly raise your entire leg up and out behind you, as high as flexibility will permit. Pay extra attention to your lower back on this one. There are many who lack adequate flexibility in this particular area.

Try to keep your leg straight and extended, and not bend at the knee. Try it even if you are only able to raise it slightly.
Finish by lowering leg back to starting position with feet together. Do one leg at a time until thoroughly exercised. Then alternate and repeat the same procedure on the other.

******************* Moving On? *******************

The exercises just given can be completed by an individual who has been inactive for a long period of time. In addition, they serve as an excellent warm up for those who seek to move on to the next stage.
If you find trouble in some or all of the previously suggested exercise movements, I recommend you seek other reading material that specifically deals with those who are altogether immobile and basically have to start over.
But if you desire more, move on to the next set of exercises in Stage II.

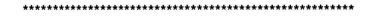

STAGE II CONDITION

1. *Deep Knee Bends* -> will again effect the muscles in legs and buttocks, emphasizing an even greater sense of balance than given earlier.

   Start in a correct standing position, with hands on hips, and feet parallel to each other about shoulder-width apart. Keep your head up and look straight ahead, then proceed to squat, bending at the knees while reaching out front with the arms for balance.

   Finish by standing up straight to original starting position, then repeat. Gradually try to reach a point where you are able to go down far enough that your legs and buttocks are at a 90 degree angle, (legs parallel with the floor). This may or may not be possible depending on one's particular physical limitations. Use your head and proceed cautiously.

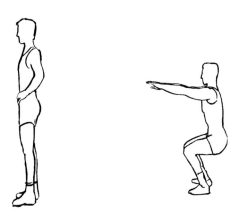

2. Another good flexibility exercise is the *Cross-Toe Touch* -> performing this exercise stimulates and stretches your hamstrings on up through your back. This is also one of the basic warm up exercises most commonly used before undergoing various sporting activities.

   First, assume the starting position of standing with arms extended straight out to the side and feet set a little wider than shoulder-width. Take one hand and bend over touching the opposite foot, then straighten back up to starting position. Repeat the same with the other hand to the opposite foot, alternating to each side as you go.

   If you are unable to touch your toe due to the lack of flexibility, take it slow and get down as far as you can without straining. If this is the case, try to at least touch your knee. Do this until you can eventually work your way down as flexibility improves.

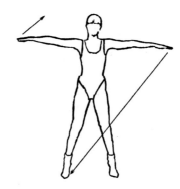

3. *Knee Push-Ups* -> will directly stimulate the chest area while indirectly affecting the shoulders, upper arms, and stomach. This is an excellent upper body exercise.

Lie face down on the floor with feet together. Place your hands a few inches wider than shoulder-width, in a line that is even with your chest.

Start by pushing yourself up until the arms are fully extended, bending only at the knees which stay on the floor. Try to keep your body in a straight line from your knees to your head.

Next, lower your body smoothly until your chest lightly touches the floor, then back up again. (Do not bounce off the floor. Always stay in control of the momentum.)

Later, when you get stronger, try the same exercise only without using your knees. Get up on your toes, yet still keeping that straight body line. Although difficult at first, using the same determination as in the previous exercises, you could very well master this one too.

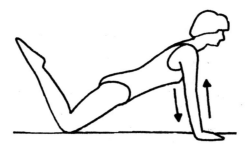

4. *Walking* -> for your health is one of the best exercises for the entire body, particularly those in the senior age group. Walking is less traumatic to the knees and joints than that of jogging or running.

Strive to get to where you can walk with enough effort to keep the heart rate up, while maintaining a safe level of physical exertion. Your objective should be to walk until there is a certain amount of muscle fatigue. (Again, since everyone is physically unique regarding shape and endurance, it would be wise to ask your doctor in determining an exercise heart rate that works best for you.) Gradually try to work your walk time up to 30 minutes or more.

5. *Power Walking* -> is simply a step up from your average walk, emphasizing a more aggressive body style (walking at a much faster pace with an emphasis on an increased and aggressive arm action). It works well as a stepping stone for those who want to someday be able to jog. But for others, power walking is all they may ever need.

6. *Dancing* -> can be a fun and enjoyable way to exercise your way to better health. Not only will it be a way to get out and meet new friends, but a good excuse to get your spouse or close friend involved in more healthy activities. Dancing provides another opportunity to share your new found health. If you prefer, regard and count each dance outing the same as you would one workout period.

7. Riding the *Stationary Bicycle* -> is very beneficial to those in the older and overweight group. This exercise not only gives you a good aerobic workout, but is an exercise that deters stress of the joints due to the non-weight-bearing effect.

8. *Cycling* -> is a favorite of many, not only due to the same reasons of the stationary bike, but those who are able, find it a nice change of pace, more scenic, and less monotonous.

9. If briskly walking for 30 or more minutes is no longer a challenge, and providing you feel up to it, then perhaps you should try *Jogging.* -> It is another excellent exercise for stimulating your whole body to better health. I find it not only just a good way to unwind physically, but mentally as well. It also provides the same benefits as walking, but at a little higher intensity level.

Therefore, it is necessary to use a bit more caution and common sense in evaluating your body's present capabilities. Endurance and increased joint stress are two examples to consider.

You should start at a slow trot (or fast walk), possibly alternating that with walking as a way to safely increase your endurance. For example, jog 3-5 minutes then walk 3-5 minutes, then back to jogging and so on. Build up slowly until you can jog continuously for 20 minutes. From then on it's up to you. You can then move at your own pace or intensity level, limited only by your own ambitions.

To help fight monotony, try choosing different routes or trails to take. Branch out, see different places and things. Try to get your neighbor or friend to jog with you. The buddy system can be safer, more challenging, and play a major role in motivation and sticking with your exercise schedule. In other words, it lessens the chance of finking out on your partner.

10. As expressed earlier in chapter 12, S*wimming ->* is one of the all time best exercises, not only for exercise in general, but also for therapeutic reasons. Swimming is used as rehabilitative therapy for many of the injured, disabled, and those who are orthopedically limited.

    Through various techniques of water training, swimming provides the muscles with a smooth, constant resistance, thus working them through a greater range of motion with less joint stress. Swimming can represent many different levels of exercise, ranging from basic full range body movements, to lap swimming, or simply treading water.

    For those whose swimming skills are questionable, or at the very least intimidating, there is now available newly designed swimming gear created especially for the water wary. These odd-shaped pieces of Styrofoam and rubber gadgets not only help you keep your head above water, but also greatly enhance the quality of your exercise periods.

    Check with your local YMCA or city recreational department for more information regarding such classes as "Water Workouts, Aquacise, or Hydro-aerobics."

11. *Sports ->* can play a major role in ones fitness training. Not only because of the quest for better health, but a great way to "play" physically. The introduction of sports into a persons lifestyle brings an added meaning to enjoying life in the later years. Sports can take on just about any form, from golf to Ping-Pong, tennis to track and field. Just ask those who are involved.

    During my Olympic training days in Southern California, I would often cross paths with seasoned veterans like Jim Vernon and Carol Johnston at many of the all-comers track meets. They both hold the world record for the pole vault in each of their own respective age groups. As difficult as it is for many to believe, they amazingly belong to the 70 and over age group, participating in probably the most difficult event in Track and Field. Both are truly inspirational and great motivators in the sense that no matter what your age, your only limits are the ones you put on yourself.

    In addition, there are many various clubs and organizations now at hand for those seniors who want to further spice up their physical activity. One such good example is the masters sports program. An organization that provides local, regional, and national competitions to men and women 40 years or older, in which you are grouped according to age and gender. For more information, contact the AAU (Amateur Athletic Union), related sites on the internet, or consult your local Adult Health Service. You can find it in your phone book.

Remember, sports for seniors are not as dangerous as inactivity. Come on, lets have some fun!

STAGE III CONDITION

Do not confuse this next group of exercises as those always more difficult than the ones previously given. If done at higher levels, some of the ones in the Stage II group also have the potential to be listed in the Stage III group, such as swimming, cycling, and so on. Again, it is all relative to you as an individual and your physical capacity.

This next particular level, I dedicate to those seniors who are in moderate to excellent shape. Those that carry little or no physical handicap, major health risks, or limitations. This level is for those who want that younger, stronger, all-around better looking body, on top of already being in good physical condition.

Make sure you have read this book entirely and understand what is involved in the outlined exercises given. Depending on your present level of fitness, many of you in the senior group may not be physically able or prepared to do some, or all of the following weight lifting exercises.

Is this or that exercise *practical* for me and my needs? Am I going to hurt myself? Ask yourself these and other pertinent questions to ensure you have chosen the proper workout strategy that best suits you and your physical capabilities.

However, it is my judgement that part of what was given earlier in regard to one exercising in their later years, bears repeating and re-emphasizing. In this case, I direct your thoughts toward the role weight-bearing exercises play upon an aging individuals bone mass, particularly those over 50.

Most who are in this age category already know the importance of basic exercise and the role it can play toward happiness and well-being. We see and hear it all the time, thanks to the various aspects of our media. But few feel the need, or at most, have failed to recognize the importance of *Strength Training* at this time in their life.

The scientific, health, and fitness communities have painstakingly researched, tested, and proven that in almost every case, EVERYONE, regardless of age, must maintain some kind of strength training regimen in order to protect that all important fundamental base, known as *structural stability*. The importance becomes magnified as each year goes by.

It doesn't mean you have to abuse yourself by lifting weights in a gym every day. No one is entering any contests here. It simply means that certain strength training exercises, like the ones in this book, if done correctly and with caution, can greatly increase ones overall present and future health rating. Hence, the final thought here is preventative maintenance.

MACHINES?

Given the choice, a free weight program takes a back seat for those in this particular group. If available, it is here I urge you to consider seeking out a nearby facility that offers a "Nautilus" or "Universal" program. If not, there are various other mechanized programs that can possibly provide you with something similar such as Cybex, Camstar, or Polaris. These programs consist of a series of specially designed exercise machines that provide the experienced, as well as the inexperienced, with a more suitable form of strength training.

These specialized programs are especially good for familiarizing one with the basic fundamentals of exercise motion, SAFELY. These types of resistance machines are convenient and easy to use. They operate in a somewhat limited range of motion and remove any chance of anything falling on you, therefore eliminating any need for a spotter.

If you are successful in locating such a facility, <u>make sure you inquire about a qualified instructor to get you started properly.</u> There is more to working these machines than meets the eye. If you do, you may find this to be just the ticket you've been looking for in a workout program, and need look no further. If this is the case, I wish you well and strongly recommend you stick with it.

If you find this is not for you, or if no such facility is available, a free weight program is perhaps now the only thing left. Follow this next workout program in the order listed but refer back to chapter nine, "Get With The Program" for the essential instructional part.

Since you will be doing each exercise only one time as suggested in the Beginners program, over time, you should strive to eventually work up to a more **circuit training** workout. That is, hitting all the major body parts one time each, per workout session, *with little or no rest between sets*.

Simply follow the given exercises in their prescribed order, moving from one to the other as quickly as your body will allow. This will enable you to get much of your (aerobic) cardiovascular training at the same time you work your muscles. Not a bad two for one, huh? The entire program shouldn't take longer than 20-30 minutes to complete.

I stress again, use your head. *Use extremely light to ZERO resistance* to begin with. Go through the motions first, BEFORE adding any resistance, and stay away from exercises that are unpractical to your needs. For this purpose, I have left out a few of those exercises which I consider high risk or unpractical for this particular age group.

Once again, <u>ALWAYS REMEMBER</u>, PROPER MOVEMENT AND TECHNIQUE IS OF MUCH MORE IMPORTANCE THAN ANY AMOUNT OF WEIGHT YOU MAY TRY USING. Lets get started.

1 SET EACH OF 8-12 REPETITIONS

(3 Days a Week)

WARM-UP
1) HALF TO THREE QUARTERS SQUATS - Optional only to those seniors who are exceptionally physically able. Otherwise this should be omitted.
2) LEG EXTENSION
3) LEG CURL
4) BENCH PRESS
5) OVERHEAD PRESS
6) TRICEP EXTENSION
7) LAT PULL-DOWN - If apparatus is available, this can be used as a substitute for Bent Over Rows.
8) INCLINE CURL
9) AB-CROSS BURN OUT - used as a substitute for the Sit-Up to reduce lower back stress.
WARM-DOWN - easy stretching, walk, or light jog.

Exercise for seniors should never be intimidating, but rather looked upon as a pleasurable experience. It should teach you to enjoy the essence of movement. For if you fail in learning to enjoy movement, you will undoubtedly drop most any exercise program you undertake.

TEENAGERS

There have been innumerable studies done, but with mixed concerns, regarding the physical training of the younger age groups. Specifically, those consisting of the pre-teen and teenagers.

We have our school systems to train the minds, but it is unfortunate that we lack the adequate follow-up on physical exercise. Without doubt, a dire necessity for developing strong healthy bodies, along with the enlightening of the spirit and further stimulation of the mind.

Therefore, the next section of this chapter is dedicated toward *educating* those youngsters in proper health and to promote an awareness of growth potential. A realization of habits they need to start forming now, to ensure a full and healthy life on down the road.

You, as a teen, at this time, have more potential for growth than you ever will again during your lifetime. That's right, *ever* in your lifetime. Physical fitness is just as, or possibly more important now, than even after you have reached adulthood.

Contrary to what some believe, good health is not something you are born with. Physical fitness is something you yourself have to develop. That's right, a **conscious** effort on your part. For good health comes not by chance or luck, but more by the way you live it.

But be aware that not everyone will develop equally. Such limiting factors as genetic makeup, motivation levels, and so on, all have their effects on the final outcome. For some, sudden growth spurts are common, while others mature much later. Therefore, don't let spirits sag by comparing yourself with others, even if the ages are the same.

The same goes with trying to estimate your true physical potential. Here, the teenage body is changing so fast that something you may have had trouble doing one day, suddenly becomes easy, with seemingly little or no effort the next. There is not much you or anyone can do to change it. This is simply a part of the maturity and hormonal changes that take place during the growth process.

All you can do is make yourself the best you can be at the time, through proper eating habits, learning proper physical exercise, and let nature take its course.

WHAT TYPE ARE YOU?

To give you somewhat of a basic idea of evaluating your present status, there is the process of "somatotyping". This is a more traditional way of assessing growth potential, by breaking down the various body types into three groups;

Ectomorph - one who is a little on the thin side with long thin bones, slightly muscled, and with low body fat.

Mesomorph - typically one with little fat, powerfully muscled, with heavy, strong bones. More commonly referred to as the "athletic" type.

Endomorph - an individual with a tendency to be more on the round, chunky side, with shorter bones and a higher percentage of body fat.

However, not every one will be able to group themselves into just one specific group. Many times, there is the overlapping of characteristics of one group into that of another. In certain instances it can become a little confusing. Regardless of what type you are, make the best of what you've got.

GIRLS ALIKE

Hey, girls, fitness training is not just for boys either, (shuffle board or badminton in P.E. class just isn't good enough). You have the same muscles that boys have, and thus an equal need for proper stimulation in growth and development. Plus the fact that you will tend to have around 10 percent more fat cells than a male in similar condition. So count yourself in.

All too often you take a back seat to the male's world of fitness. Why? Who knows. Perhaps it's the larger emphasis male sports seems to play, or maybe it's the relentless uphill fight of traditional gender stereotypes. Whatever the case may be, it doesn't matter. What does matter, is that you go out and stake your own claim in this modern age of fitness. The teenage years are difficult enough without having to worry about the added pressures of obesity and insecurity.

OK, so you do exercise, but are leery of picking up the tempo, fearing unlady like consequences such as weight gain, muscle mass, or all around size increases. It's misconceptions like these that become common when discussing topics like weight training for females and a big reason why many tend to shy away from such activity.

Well, forget it. For the most part, you should have little worry about getting over-muscular due to the decreased absence of necessary muscle-building hormones (testosterone). Girls should know, that unlike boys, physically, it is nearly impossible to build a *large* amount of muscle mass naturally. Feel better?

However, with persistence and determination, it IS possible to increase a discrete amount of muscle size and definition, in the effort to emphasize a well-toned and proportioned figure. After all, what girl would turn down the supreme opportunity to be able to finally have that rare, killer figure? So what do you say ladies, are you in or out?

Nevertheless, in or out, male OR female, as a teen it is never too late to change yourself. Your present structure of bone, muscle, and fat, CAN and WILL be changed with proper diet and exercise. Although changes can still be made when you reach your twenties, thirties, and so on, never to the extent to what you can accomplish in your adolescent years.

PUMPING IRON - TAKE CARE!

Just a quick reminder before going any further, not every type of exercise that you see, hear, or read is good for you at every age. Just because Joe Bodybuilder does it, doesn't mean it's the right thing for you. Granted, certain muscle magazines, videos, and bodybuilding programs play a big part in the overall education process, but often times overemphasize heavy training practices. It is here you must be careful and avoid *heavy* weight training. It's a common mistake most teens make in the beginning. Not only are the young bones still in the fragile growing process, but it also takes considerable time and patience to learn proper training techniques that become nothing short, of essential.

Given this, the number one recommendation to the true beginner is to try and gain access to such circuit training programs like "Nautilus" or "Universal" as advised earlier in this chapter. They offer the beginner a safe, non-confusing outlook on working out. The resistance can be changed merely by pulling a pin and does not require a spotter. They help avoid cheating and decrease the risk of injury over that of free weights.

If used correctly, such machines will safely work each body part through it's full range of motion, with the added benefit of also working the cardiovascular system. A choice approved by most physicians and in my opinion, perfect for beginners through all ages. But unfortunately, and all to often, this type of equipment is many times unavailable in your area as well as unpractical for the home.

This now limits the choices to that of free-form exercises. Calisthenics work well for starters, with which you replace some of the barbell exercises with that of your own body weight. Some examples include push-ups, chair dips, sit-ups, chin-ups, deep knee bends, and jumping jacks, just to name a few.

But it is the free weight portion of this book, combined with good eating habits and aerobics that offers the most versatility with that of practicality. As you will soon find, free weight training involves a whole new form of discipline regarding body control, body response, and visual effects.

Such programs build strength and symmetry by developing not only the major muscle groups themselves, but also those peripheral supporting muscles as well. This, in addition to following instructions *to the letter*, will enable you to feel, as well as see, your newly discovered potential. Here is what you do;

Simply follow as instructed, the beginner or intermediate programs in chapter nine, "Get With The Program."

It will be tough at first, no doubt about it. Especially when learning to control that perfect rhythm, technique, and balance that is required. Here, difficulty and frustration is likely, while patience and persistence will be the key. All must quickly realize that results take time. Actually, quite a long time. This trial and error process we must all go through is often long and arduous. Experience will prove some areas develop easier than others. The stubborn spots only mean you have found an area that needs special attention, and therefore more work.

For you athletes participating in sports and/or other extra curricular activities, it's obvious that you will require a higher level of fitness training in order to excel above and beyond. Quite simply, more cardiovascular endurance, more flexibility, and more strength.

Finally, *DON'T FORGET* the importance of setting personal goals. Draw clear, precise pictures in your mind, never stopping until they have been reached. Ask yourself such things as, what exactly do you want to accomplish? At what level of strength or activity do you strive? Which is more important, getting a good workout in, or goofing off, going to a party, or watching TV? Above all, will you do what it takes?

PRE-TEENS

This pre-teen group consists of the twelve-year-olds down through preschool. If you are a pre-teenage youngster or a parent of one, after reading up to this point you now know how important it is to develop proper fitness habits at an early age. To me, the recommendation is simple, STAY ACTIVE and HAVE FUN!

Parents, encourage your child to try different things, be supportive of extra-curricular activities, and keep them **physically active**. It all begins with you. You should lead by example through positive attitudes, positive lifestyles, and through proper exercise and eating habits. All these factors form a much needed molding process that will in every way affect their present and future outlook on life in general.

Again, the buzz word here is **"PLAY"**. Because variety at any age, is without a doubt, the key to continued exercise happiness. Children that play a lot tend to have better coordination skills, higher energy levels, better dispositions, handle stress situations better in or out of the family, and are better adapted in learning to interact with their fellow playmates (such as sharing, camaraderie, and competition).

Therefore, a child should not be put on any specific "workout program" per se. A kid should be allowed to be kid, do what kids do, without the added pressure of maintaining a pre-set, scheduled workout program. During this time in a child's life, the attention span is low and the frustration level is high. This is probably the only time in which they will be able to have that care-free, happy-go-lucky feeling. Allow them to simply enjoy!

Let there be no misunderstanding, organized little league, soccer, or taking Karate lessons are all great. But not to the point the child stops having fun due to increased pressure from his or her playmates, coaches, or even their own parents.

Always encourage, but never push!

INVEST IN LIFE

In conclusion, and perhaps looking at the whole picture from a different perspective, a little extra effort in proper long term exercise practices could conceivably be thought of as *investments* toward <u>future</u> health and well being. Investments not only for the moment, but for much later on down the road. It's a time when all your previous habits, good or bad, eventually come into play.

For throughout our lives, we constantly work and plan for our future. We work hard, day after day, week after week, year after year, hoping one day it will all pay off. A fraction of us even go one step further and set aside a little money as an investment for the retired years. A time that is looked upon as worry-free and fun loving. Yet, with all the planning and forethought that is applied, seldom does one consider the prime investment of all.

Your Health! .... What condition will it be in, long after those working years are over?

Sadly, there are still too many out there that finally come to realize the importance of proper health and maintenance much too late in life. Yes, I am again emphasizing the point of staying active, but in this instance, pointing the finger directly at exercise. Exercise should also be thought of as an investment. An investment for the future.

Try dabbling with the thought of exercise as a belated gift or hard-earned currency. An investment that accrues over time for those who earn it. Let's also say, that for every hour of exercise you put in now, **could be equal to an <u>extra day</u> of prime health and happiness later on.** Sort of like saving up sick days for a lifetime, to start using or cashing in when you hit those senior years. A time that still matters. A time that can be all you want it to be.

Although the proof behind this way of thinking is impossible to actually document, it is more the frame of mind one must have to get up and get things started, as well as consistently maintain throughout. So start making that investment in exercise. Every time you do, you'll be making an investment in life!

CHAPTER FOURTEEN:

HANG IN THERE!

Congratulations! You are now on track to a new and healthier lifestyle. One that will provide you with a firm, toned, shapely body, bursting with health that both looks and feels great. All end products of a successful diet/exercise program. All one has to remember is the Big "3".

STEP ONE: **WISE UP!**

Get checked out by your doctor, discard any and all unhealthful habits, and <u>become more knowledgeable</u> on future health and lifestyle changes.

STEP TWO: **BECOME NUTRITIONALLY SOUND**

Practice healthy eating, with *balanced* meals that contain less fats.
(*Chapter 4, Food and Fast Food Reference Guides*)

STEP THREE: **JUST SAY YES TO EXERCISE**

Improve body composition, firm, shape, and tone muscles, through weight training.
(*Chapters 9 & 10*)

Increase your metabolic rate and burn additional calories through endurance exercise.
(*Chapter 12*)

Regardless of what your primary objectives may have been in the beginning, always know that each of the Big "3" should play just as important a role towards complete fitness as the other. All should be considered a package deal with each given equal effort and attention to detail. Understand it! Follow it! Do it! And you can't go wrong!

****

And now, to help you bring this book to a conclusion, I am leaving you with these final concepts so as to leave no stone overturned. Most definitely, the fewer the stumbling blocks, the faster one attains ones own *Physical Results*.

****

ADAPTATIONAL CAPABILITIES

Eventually, at some point on the exercise highway, both the novice and experienced will have to learn to develop *adaptational capabilities*. That is, the ability to change, or recognize the need for change, during this or any other workout program. This is very important.

There will come a time when your *body* will not respond to a certain exercise or workout routine in the same way it used to, leaving you stale and unsatisfied.

Likewise, there will come a time when your *mind* will become numb, when feelings of boredom or burn-out set in and begin to negatively affect the outcome of your workout. In either case, one must learn to keep things as interesting and productive as possible.

Over time, learn to experiment with different techniques or different variations of exercise instead of the same old thing. Twist the wrist a little more on this one, or move the arm a little differently here and there. You could add a workout partner, or extra exercises for your favorite body parts. Perhaps change the times in which you work out each day, or even the gym location itself. Try different atmospheres, different kinds of music, and so forth.

The possibilities are not as limited as some may think, although much can only be learned through experience. I think a fellow by the name of Dan Stanford said it best when he said, *"Experience is what you get when you don't get what you want"*.

YOU ARE ONLY HUMAN

Experience will also teach you that even with the best possible program, you must accept if you haven't already, that not every workout will be upbeat and perfect. As you will soon find, there will be times when you've reached a sort of exercise high, feeling as

214

if you have just conquered the world. But just the same, there will be other times when you will feel beat and somewhat depressed, unable to meet your expectations, feeling as though nothing has been accomplished.

No matter what anyone says, how hard you try, or manage to change things up, there will most certainly be episodes when you feel as though little or no progress has been made. It happens to each and every one of us at one time or another. Not surprisingly, this is quite normal and should be accepted as something that comes with the territory.

For it is during these down times, when our true character and inner strength that runs deep in each of us, *must come out* and pull us through. In other words, don't give up! No matter how difficult it seems, know that you MUST keep it going, tomorrow, the next day, and into the next. Remind yourself that no matter how you feel at the time or what your present frame of mind is, there most definitely will be better days ahead. Remember, you're only human.

PLAY TIME

A part of human nature is to have fun. In this instance, fitness and sports are most often thought of and viewed as one, that of combining a skill with true physical talent. It's no wonder that those who regularly compete in various sporting activities find it easier to stick with their exercise program, than those of their counterparts who do not. In essence, sports seem to break up the effort of exercise while providing further incentive to excel.

Moreover, those who actively engage in various sporting activities almost automatically find, that sooner or later, their level of desire and motivational drive expand and grow, in order to meet new goals and expectations.

Sporting activities, whether competitive or not, are an excellent way to reap and enjoy those healthy benefits you have worked so hard for. It is here, I urge all to find a sport that can be enjoyed now and forever, yet, with the assurance of still being able to work it in and around your present exercise program. After all, what better way is there to "play physically?"

COUNT YOUR BLESSINGS

While some of us work or play our way towards making ourselves better, others are not as fortunate. Therein lies the shame, a regrettable contingency of why so many Americans still continue to talk themselves out of starting some kind of exercise program, either because they believe themselves to be too fat, too old, or just plain too far out of shape.

However, I find most of the time, those excuses have no backing, and more often than not, come down to being just plain lazy.

215

Sadly, these types of individuals seem to take what they have for granted, in turn, never fully realizing their true potential. Their true happiness.

If this is you, look around! There are those among us right now, right this instant, that would give anything for the opportunity to build a better and healthier body, but due to circumstances beyond their control, will never have that chance. At least not in the same sense you and I may envision.

Take note of those unfortunate few that began life, or acquired beyond their control, certain strikes against them. I am speaking of those with various birth defects, diseases, or victims of crippling accidents. Many such handicapped individuals struggle just to survive, and yet some go on to achieve the impossible, accomplishing feats of physical skill and endurance that most of us with normal capabilities would never consider. These amazing individuals continue to prove to be an inspiration to us all, *accepting reality, not excuses*! If they can do it with their limitations, **then so can you**!

So, before you put a lot of effort into trying to think up a sound excuse for not exercising, think of what you do have and be thankful. Get off your duff and do something. Unlike the unfortunate few, you DO have a choice, DON'T WASTE IT!

LUCK, THERE'S NO SUCH THING

After reading to this point, whether you are getting ready to start this particular program or have already begun, I DO NOT wish you luck. That's right, I'll say it again. I wish you no luck what-so-ever. Because when it comes to exercise, living and eating right, there is no such thing as luck.

Luck is for those *waiting* for a break, one that usually never comes. Luck is for those unfortunate individuals that achieve little in life, always waiting for opportunities to come to them with little or no obligation on their part. A proverbial attitude of always having their needs and wants "served on a silver platter".

It is the *doers* that will eventually succeed. No matter what the handicap, doers will *make* and *create* their own breaks, overcoming obstacles both great and small.

To reach a state of complete fitness, and yet be able to maintain it throughout the rest of your lifetime will be one of your most important obstacles to conquer. To what degree of difficulty this obstacle becomes, will depend entirely upon you and how hard you make it for yourself. Be a DO'ER. Regain control, over you, your body, your destiny. DO IT and DO IT NOW!

PARTING THOUGHTS

In closing, I commend anyone that possesses the will to undertake **any** kind of exercise program for the pursuit of better health and well being. Whether it's the housewife out for her 30 minute daily walk or the dedicated bodybuilder settling in to his

216

normal two and a half hour weight lifting ritual. Regardless of who, or how long, it can at times be a hard choice to make, and actually doing it can be even harder.

But, it's individuals like you that make this big world go around. The lifestyle foundation we so carefully lay down today, will be the format from which our future will evolve tomorrow. Issues such as health care, child development, and standard of living will largely depend upon how you take care of yourself. In other words, just what kinds of seeds are you sowing, for yourself, as well as the impact you have upon those around you? Think about this very seriously for a moment!

Also, it is my sincere hope that every person who reads this book will be able to capture the energy and enthusiasm that continually dwells within me, much of which comes from enjoying an active and fit lifestyle, with the added optimism of further encouraging and promoting fitness for others. A challenge if you will, from me to you, to any and all, to those who demand *physical results.*

As I mentioned before, I am not going to wish you luck, but I will say this, I wish you well, now and into the future, and look forward knowing more and more of you will be leading healthier, happier, more productive lives. **NEVER** give up, **ALWAYS** remain positive, and above all, **HANG IN THERE!**

IF YOU WANT IT, YOU <u>CAN</u> HAVE IT, PERIOD!

ABOUT THE AUTHOR

I grew up on a fifth generation family farm in South Central Kansas, with my parents and three younger brothers. I graduated from Haven High, a small town high school 8 miles from home, then continued on through college at Fort Hays State University to graduate with a bachelor's degree in Animal Science. From there, I ventured to Southern California for five years to train for the 1984 and 1988 Olympic teams. Now, I'm back home continuing to farm full time as well as working full time for a nearby city as a firefighter/EMT.

For years I often pondered why failure remains such a common place in our world of fitness, given the vast library of information, instruction and incentives right at our fingertips. Up until ten years ago, I had always been in the arena but never took note as a spectator, that is, until now!

It is here I feel a need to somehow connect with you, the reader, the despondent fitness wanna-be, the average every day exercise buff, the prospective athlete, weekend warrior, and all the other desperate souls vainly searching for answers, by exposing the often times, discouraging, but normal set-backs that occur as part of the overall fitness trek. It is my sincere hope that this brief account and background familiarization of my own trials and tribulations in climbing the fitness ladder will lead you to a better understanding of how the world of health and fitness has influenced and guided me to what I am today, along with the unique opportunities and achievements that I've come away with as a result.

For I truly consider myself just an average guy with above average goals, carrying a strong desire to do my best in whatever I want or do. Granted, in many ways I've been luckier than most. The gift of being born healthy surrounded by complete family support is probably the most important jump-start to health there is, but for the most part, it's been a struggle like anything else. Yes, I CAN relate to the normal day-to-day challenges and know how hard it can be to reach any measurable degree of fitness. But, if I can make things happen through living a fit and healthy lifestyle, then I truthfully feel anyone can. Nothing fancy or overly complicated, just the basics.

FROM THE BEGINNING

As a youngster, I was pretty much your average, energetic kid, with average skills. I was never one of the lucky few blessed with raw natural talent to do many things. Quite honestly, I was more of a hard worker than a fast learner.

What I did have in my corner was an enormous amount of family support. My brothers and I were lucky to have parents that always encouraged us to do our best, but never pushed. They were ALWAYS there for us during our triumphs, as well as our failures. It didn't matter whether if it was in sports, school, studies, or band.

I matured like any other youngster, growing and learning by my mistakes. Like most teenagers, it wasn't until high school that my individuality began to take shape.

During high school, I lettered in most of the major sports, made the honor roll, and was honored by being voted into several different royalties. I was also active in various other school functions, which led me to being selected to the national publication of "WHO'S WHO AMONG AMERICAN HIGH SCHOOL STUDENTS."

WORKING OUT

It was around the end of my senior year in high school that I started to learn more about weight training and fitness. Up until this time, I thought I knew just about everything there was to know about the subject. After all, I had been active in all major sports, accompanied by a multitude of various other workout programs since I was in 7th grade. But my wake-up call abruptly came when my brother and I began taking evening Karate lessons. It was a time when things finally started coming together.

Initially, we were put in a weight room in the back of the dojo first, before setting one foot in our Karate class. I vividly remember these huge guys handing us barbells with pre-selected weights, instructing us on what exercises to do.

However, I was a little disheartened by the fact that I must have appeared not quite as strong as I myself believed. The weights they gave me were considerably less than what I was normally used to using. So naturally, I felt the need to clue them in on what I believed to be the proper poundage. I was stronger than that and not the total rookie they may have thought. Their reply was a stern look, a cracked smile, and a firm answer of....... DO IT! Reluctantly, I respected their authority and experience and proceeded to follow their lead, yet with the attitude, "I'll show 'em."

BREAKTHROUGH

At first, the resistance felt way too easy. I didn't think I was going to get anywhere this way. I didn't want to be one to say *I told you so*......... then WHAMMO, that's when it happened. I couldn't believe the burn I was getting. They were right! You could almost see the muscles pop right in front of your eyes. It was amazing. I had never before felt anything like it.

That whole next day, I was so stiff and sore, I could barely drink a glass of water or even reach back far enough to scratch my back. But did this change my outlook? Did this make me want to quit or go back to the old way? No way! On the contrary, I welcomed these new feelings of accomplishment, looking upon the stiff and sore sensations as a positive step towards a new level. Solid proof that I had somehow reached a major breakthrough I didn't even know was possible.

Needless to say, it wasn't easy surviving track practice, weight workouts, and the Karate classes immediately afterward for those first few weeks. But I did survive and came to realize just how forgiving my body could be.

A MASTERS' INFLUENCE

A short time later, I came upon an early book by Arnold Schwarzenegger, which later proved to be yet another tool of inspiration. It provided me with more variations in exercise, leading me to develop my own program, catering to my own needs and personal goals.

In addition to his outward physical prominence, you could almost feel his strong, positive mental attitude come right out and grab you. A trait he is also famous for. It was not until a few years later, that I really began to understand the importance of using the mind in just such a positive manner. I had always heard or read of such people who could give themselves that extra edge, in all things like sports, business, careers, and so on, but never thought it would ever pertain to me. I found it to be something with which you cannot totally get from a book, but only through experiencing yourself.

GETTING SERIOUS

While studying in college, I chose to continue my athletics in Track and Field, where I became a 3-Time All American pole vaulter. I also continued to train for the Decathlon and Karate simultaneously.

In each case, I had set my goals high, with the known fact that I must carefully and systematically increase my work load in order to achieve each one. If I expected my body to do more, I had to give it more, but finding the time to do it would be the hard part.

Actually, when all was said and done, there were few options open for a hard working, full time farm boy. Although what followed was tough and demanding, it somehow got done.

I worked on the farm by day to financially support myself for each upcoming year of college, while training in the evenings to develop my strength and flexibility for each upcoming track season. I would work all day and quit a little early, somewhere around 9 or 10 p.m. Then you could find me down in the basement hitting the weights for 1 1/2 hours of solid, intense workouts, six nights a week.

Most of the time after working all day, I found myself so exhausted, working out was the last thing I wanted to do. (Sound familiar?) Then there were times I was OK physically, but shot down mentally, simply, downright burned out on exercise altogether. So many times, all I wanted to do was take a break, do something different, go out with my friends, play a little kill ball with my brothers (that's barefoot basketball with no rules), do anything but this. I clearly remember searching for any, that's right, ANY legitimate excuse to skip just one measly workout.

Did I ever? Not hardly. Rarely was there an excuse sound enough to justify skipping at any time, (except of course barring a funeral, major holiday, or heaven forbid, the promising lure of summer wheat harvest!) Somehow, some way, I was always able to force myself to jump right in and get it done. That's right, just get it done! Back then, I found that every time I could conquer anything negative regarding my workouts, my mind as well as my body would grow that much stronger. Realizing this was never something that openly jumped up out of the blue and bit me, instead, it was something that gradually sneaked up on me over a period of time.

From that point on I soon began to realize just how vital it had become to keep my goals, not only clear and focused, but ruggedly consistent as well.

The sacrifice and discipline that was required during that period in my life instilled in me the importance of doing what it takes to reach a specific goal, whether it meant getting a diploma, or achieving All-American status. There would soon come a time when I would find that all my past training and determination would eventually be put to the test.

GOING FOR THE GOLD

After graduating from college in 1983 and with strong support from my family, I decided to postpone any career plans and try out for the 1984 Olympic team. I felt I was talented enough to continue my athletic career, thus putting to use those previous years of training and preparation. Here again, was an example of an average guy striving to reach something just a little bit higher than anyone else, a goal most felt unattainable.

Why not? I had nothing to lose from at least trying. So what if it was a long shot. It was there right in front of me, a lifetime opportunity I just couldn't turn down. There was nothing else at that time that could replace or dampen the excitement that was building inside me.

Rapidly, I was becoming driven. My mind was so pumped to the thought of making the team, I could visualize nothing else. I guess I had what is commonly referred to as "tunnel vision", driving those around me crazy. It was a point whereby I chose my goal, focused toward it on a straight and narrow line, and went for it! All the while, my little voice inside was constantly reminding me that in whatever I choose to do, do it right and go all out. Hold to that commitment, never quitting or stopping halfway.

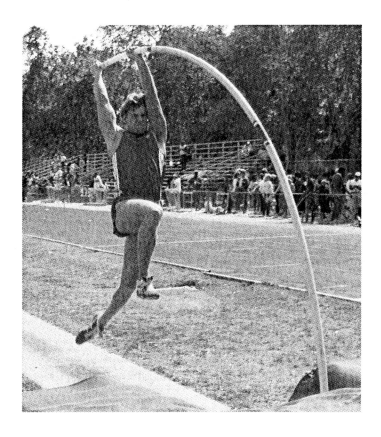

After exploring all the angles and options available, I knew it was time to make some big decisions. I knew I was going to give the Olympics a try, that had already been decided. But, in order for me to stand the best chance of success, I would require an atmosphere with consistently good weather, good coaching, proper facilities, and numerous competitions. Nothing around home had that. Running wind sprints down country roads or pole carries in a plowed up field just wasn't going to do it. It was at that point I decided to temporarily move to Los Angeles, the mecca of Track and Field.

Once there, I worked various full and part-time jobs to support myself, then trained 2-3 hours after work, six days a week. I had a "pedal-to-the-metal, no-holds-barred" attitude. I had never pushed myself as hard as I did then.

Well, to make a long story short, it turned out that I failed to make the 1984 Olympic team that year. Although there were no regrets or excuses, I did give it my best shot. But at the same time, I also came away feeling unfulfilled. I felt like I was just starting to put the pieces together to being one of the nations best. I had come so far and had already invested much time and effort. If I only had more time.

ROUND TWO

After discussing it with my family, I made an even bigger decision, in that I wanted to attempt the 1988 Olympic team bound for Seoul, Korea. That meant four more years of hardship, grueling training schedules, and much sacrifice. Big time Track and Field was still new to me and I still enjoyed it. But more importantly, it was something I needed to do for myself. Deep down, I knew if I quit now I would never forgive myself later on. I had to see just how far I could go.

During those next four years my mental strength grew tenfold. That's right, grew. But it wasn't due to the many successes and triumphs as one might first think. This was no small town boy coming from behind and making it big story here. In reality, the low points far outnumbered the highs. So many failures, frustrations, and setbacks, I don't think anyone would have thought less of me if I had given up and thrown in the towel at that point.

But I didn't! Somehow, someway, I stubbornly picked myself up and tried again and again. For every time I would have a bad practice, or encounter some kind of training block, I would strive to focus full attention on that particular problem, then work and push until I would eventually prevail. I would accept nothing else.

No sooner would I overcome one technical problem when another would surface and set me back again.

Is my approach off? No, my plant is all wrong. Maybe I'm not getting enough knee drive into the pit. Should I go to a bigger pole? How about getting vertical?.......no, that's not a problem. Speed? Well, I'm doing the best that I can with what the good Lord gave me. And on and on.

This compounding frustration along with miscellaneous injuries, and the pressure I would put on myself to perform, made my training increasingly difficult by the day. I was steadily becoming emotionally drained and burned out. Often I asked why I was putting myself through this. Is it worth all this just to fly through the air over a bar? I missed my family and longed for my beloved farm, nevertheless I continued on relentlessly.

Although this emotional up and down roller coaster was getting to me, something inside said to keep trying, just do your best. Never do anything half way or quit anything until it is finished. So without trying to sound like a broken record, I put my forehead into the wind, adjusted accordingly, and pushed on.

Surprisingly, as the days turned into weeks, and weeks into months, every setback brought even MORE determination. My mind and willpower continued to grow stronger and stronger each day. Seldom was there a time I was unable to pull something positive out of a negative situation. A process of mental conditioning that I learned to use both on and off the track. A valuable lesson that carried me through the toughest of times then, and now.

NOT IN THE CARDS

Well, I missed making the team again. Sorry, but there is no storybook ending here. No red, white, and blue fanfare or Olympic theme playing in the background. No hometown parades or big buck endorsement contracts. Truthfully, I was more than delighted to finally have it over with, BUT more importantly, I have no regrets what-so-ever having given it my best effort. I tried, and that says a lot, for me anyway, and that's what really counts. I never would have known, and always would have wondered for the rest of my life of "what could have been". I feel very fortunate to have had the opportunity to chase a dream, whatever the outcome might be.

With this, I have since learned to never again miss any opportunity, or neglect pursuing any goal or dream that happens to come my way. For life is composed of many such challenges and one should never be afraid to take their shot when it comes along. No one!

OPEN DOORS

Although I failed to make the team, I reaped many other side benefits from the unique experience. Many other doors seemed to open up, side doors mainly. It was almost as if all I had to do was honestly try and put forth an effort and something positive would come out of it, *even if that something had nothing to do with the initial goal.*

For instance, while training in Los Angeles, I made many good friends and had many unforgettable experiences. I will always hold in my memory the honor of being associated with, and having competed against, some of the best in the world.

I also managed to acquire a Hollywood agent and did a few television commercials. Friends also encouraged me to try a little modeling on the side. I didn't like the modeling, it just wasn't me. But for this country farm boy, doing national/international television commercials was a great experience in itself. After all, how many Kansas farmers are members of The Screen Actors Guild?

But, above all, I learned more about myself. What my body can and can't do. Mentally, how strong can I get? How far can I go, in anything I choose or desire?

ONWARD AND UPWARD

Looking back, I have found that the ups and downs experienced in day to day life are much the same as in Olympic training. Whereas no sooner do you conquer one problem, when another one pops up. It is a continuous process that keeps life from being humdrum and monotonous, always reminding you of its constant challenges. After all, it is such challenges as these that will either force you to back down, **or force you to grow.**

225

Yet, always bear in mind, no one is immune to failure. Not you or anyone else. Enduring such adversity should lead to a strengthening of character and body, not weakness or ridicule. But this can only happen if you remain positive, decipher where and why you have failed, and learn from it (don't do it again). Walter Wriston, former chairman of Citicorp said it another way: "Failure is not a crime. Failure to learn from failure is."

I, too, have since learned to treat each failure merely as a stepping stone, a unique and memorable lesson **toward** success. It's a concept each and every one of us must learn to accept and believe from this point forward. For it is **you** who must be strong and solid enough within yourself, to successfully handle what life dishes out. Again, only YOU and no one else.

It is with this thought that I give you this book, in hopes that if you are shown a way in which to control your mind and body through *diet* and *exercise*, that you too, will be better able to control the reality of life's many surprises (failures), and fruits waiting to be reaped.

JUST AND AVERAGE GUY

I'm (obviously) no Arnold Schwartznegger or Jane Fitness U.S.A. I'm no movie star or famous athlete. I pretend to be no one but myself, enjoying most everything I do while living life to its fullest. I handle and control my own destiny, through hard work, dedication, and perseverance. I believe the pleasures of which life have to offer are to be savored and enjoyed.

BUT, one rarely gets something for nothing and initially requires some kind of effort on your part. Becoming physically fit is no different. I am just an average guy, trying to share with others a successful way to achieve their physical aspirations.

Here, I truly hope you find inner happiness and a sense of personal strength through the dedicated efforts of this book. Thank you!

Remember, the ***path*** up the mountain, is of more value than just sitting atop the summit. –Brad Nachtigal

3-Time All-American Pole Vaulter
2-time Olympic Hopeful
TV Commercial Actor
Part-Time Model
Personal Fitness Instructor
5th Generation Farmer
Firefighter\EMT
Height: 6'0"
Weight: 180 lbs.
Body Fat: 6%

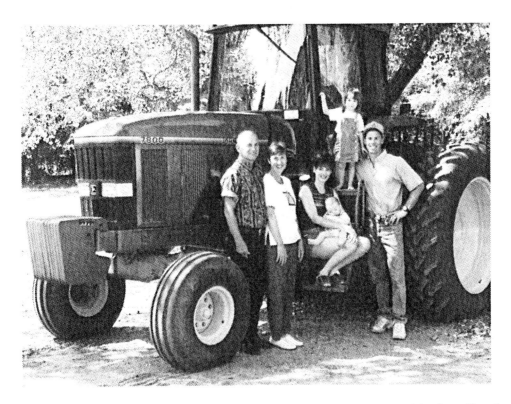

The Nachtigal's from left to right: Roy, Ann, Angie, Cade, Haylee, Brad

TROUBLESHOOTING: "1-800-HELP!"

Having trouble with a particular exercise? Not getting where you want or feel what you think you should? Perhaps, you desire more than what is provided. Well, you're in the right place.

While there is no one exercise program, book or instructional video out on the market today that has the capability to zero in on each individual's exercise problems, this, may be as close as you'll ever get. This self-guided troubleshooting section resembles a customer service 800 line, but instead of dialing a phone for help, you simply turn here. A unique method of problem solving right at your own fingertips.

Hopefully, this self-sufficient approach will be more successful in pushing just the right buttons towards stimulating both mind and body. Often, one responds completely different when instructed in a slightly altered fashion. Invariably, it all comes down to using a different word, different gesture, or different mind-set to attain that sometimes illusive, mind- blowing, body-burning feeling of accomplishment. All suggestions are specialized tricks-of-the-trade, compiled from years of exercise experience and a goodly amount of trial and error.

WARNING

Use this section sparingly and ONLY when needed. Otherwise, confusion and frustration is likely, especially for beginners.

"Troubleshooting" is to be used ONLY as a reference guide to pin- pointing and solving problems associated with a specific weight training exercise as outlined here in this book.

In other words, turn here **only when you are well into your Program, and at one time or another, feel like you are getting no where with any one particular exercise, THEN is the time to refer back here and find out what you are doing wrong.**

Envision it sort of like being able to reach for a road map in the event you ever get lost or side-tracked. One that will allow you to reach your final destination quickly and efficiently, while avoiding all detours and wrong ways that could possibly lead you astray.

TAKING IT STEP-BY-STEP

Simply locate **only** the exercise you are having difficulty with, then try each suggestion one at a time, always beginning with the first one. I say again, *one at a time*.

Do not attempt to comprehend the entire listing all at once. In other words, read the first suggestion and give it a try. If it makes a difference and helps you out, even a little, stop there and read no further. But if needed, keep going until you find one that makes a difference.

Remember, it is up to you to determine how much you are able to get out of this program by making sure you follow as per instructed.

One more time, *as per instructed*. For when one provides you with a tool to make a job more efficient, make sure the job gets done right by using it the way it was intended!

<u>*TROUBLESHOOTING*</u> <u>Weight Training Rule Of Thumb</u>

Generally, the more demanding you can make each movement, each motion, or each maneuver, the more productive that technique becomes.

BENCH PRESS

- Concentrate! *Mentally* feel the first rep through the last. Rely only on the pectoral muscles to get the weight up on each rep, rather than relying too much on your arms. Isolate!

- Avoid bouncing the bar off the chest area in an attempt to initiate or use any momentum in getting it back up. Each repetition should be as smooth and in control as possible. Bouncing may indicate too much weight is being used. If so, drop it!

- Be consciously aware of the role negative resistance plays each time the bar is *lowered*, in turn, zeroing in on the actual *sensations* involved during a full and complete stretch of your pectorals. In other words, don't just let the weight drop each time. Stay in complete control from start to finish.

- Check to make sure you are going the full range of motion on each rep, yet, stopping just before full locking of the elbows. Never go only half way.

- Are you flexing your pecs at the top end of each repetition? You will notice additional stimulation plus faster results when this is done.

- Are you using too much resistance? More times than not, this is usually the biggest problem.

  If you are, it will more than likely steal your concentration from your technique. Thus, you end up over-straining, shifting, and contorting your body all out of position just to get the weight back to the up position. In turn, you will loose form, the proper feel, and prolong your desired results.

- Drop the weight to the point you can perform the bench press *technically correct for at least the first 6 or 8 reps of each set.* (Refer to Chapter 7, "Take It Off!") Then try it again.

- Make sure the bar is consistently brought down to the nipple area of the chest, not any lower or any higher on the body.

- Always maintain a consistent and efficient center of thrust.

- Keep the bar moving. Avoid resting too long between reps. Just give the pecs a short flex at the top, then back down you go again.

- If you continue to have problems isolating your pecs either physically or mentally, check to make sure you are not allowing your elbows drift too close to your side. Allowing this to happen tends to divert some of the emphasis from the chest and put more pressure on the shoulders.

  Keep the elbows pointed out, always away from your sides, *from beginning to end.*

- If available, some prefer to seek out additional stimulation by using a further specialized incline or decline bench apparatus. (The incline option usually comes with most of todays multi-use benches.)

  Due to the different degree of balance required, it is recommended for only those that carry a little more experience. But if the desire and skills are there, go for it! Such variations of the Bench Press all provide an additional fulfillment to this particular area of the body.

- Check your hand grip. You may experience varied results by moving your grip slightly in or out.

  For instance, using a narrow shoulder-with grip, or even closer, seems to work well when other things don't. However, you generally have to use a lighter amount of weight.

- Never grip the bar too tight. Over-gripping steals concentration from where it is needed.

  Instead, increase your pectoral concentration by only gripping the bar tight enough to stay secure. The most comfortable position is usually with the bar resting across the heal of the hands.

- Make sure to use proper breathing technique. You should inhale smoothly as you lower the weight down and exhale when ramming it up.

  If you still have trouble, it helps to inhale deeply first, before you begin the actual movement of each lift. This will ensure yourself enough lung capacity to be able to exhale properly, thus making for more of a controlled and coordinated effort.

- If all else has failed up to this point, you can now try adding a little more weight resistance to this exercise.

HORIZONTAL DUMBBELL FLYE

- **Concentrate**! Mentally crawl into the pectoral muscles themselves. You are their master. You control every fiber that makes them function. Stay focused.

- Sometimes it helps to create a mental picture of visualizing the arms only as *solid, fixed levers* on which the weights are attached. This type of mental imaging often helps in forcing only the pecs to do the actual work.

- Be sure to go through the fullest range of motion possible, but always with caution, never going past the point of extreme pain or present physical capability.

- Try holding the fully stretched position for a short one count on the bottom of each rep. Feel the stretch? Now bring it back up and feel the isolation. Now keep it going.

- Imagine *hugging* or squeezing a large round tree, as if the trunk were so large you were barely able to bring both hands together on the other side.

  This crude, mental crutch, if you will, should help you maintain the proper wide circle of motion technique, rather than that of a pressing movement.

- Always check to make sure you are maintaining proper exercise technique. You will find that the more fatigued you become during this exercise, the more difficult it becomes to prevent the elbows from over-bending, in an effort to finish the last couple repetitions during each respective set. In other words, they bend too much. This then becomes more of a pressing motion than a wide circle flye.

  This is **only** acceptable when pushing yourself to finish the very end of the set, as long as the first 75% of the set is flawless. If you break form **too early** in any one particular set, you have added on too much weight. Take it off!

- Double check your body positioning during exercise. Keep the buttocks on the bench at all times and feet flat on the floor. If either of these two are not right, then you are using too much weight.

- Are you flexing at the *top* end of each rep? In failing to do so, you are probably missing out on <u>half</u> of the stimulation and gain possible. Try holding each top end flex, for a short one count. Then back down and repeat.

- Another method related to flexing, is to think about firmly pressing the dumbbells together the moment they come together at the top, as if you are mentally trying to crush them between your hands.

(A prime example of how one could perform a self-test on what one should actually experience and feel during this exercise, would be to refer back to chapter 7, on the *Flex* method.)

- Mentally, go one step further and visualize yourself being able to keep an imaginary quarter on edge, tightly tucked in the center of the chest during the top end flexing process. Work on giving it a good squeeze on each rep.

- Another little trick of the trade is to slightly rotate your wrists inward as they come together at the top, as if you are trying to touch the outside heel of each hand. That should probably do it.

- Are you unable to understand why you only feel like half of your chest is being worked on this exercise? It may be because the same principle holds true here as in the Bench Press. You must keep the dumbbells in a **consistent** area over the chest in which you start and finish each rep.

  If you finish each top-end rep with the dumbbells over your head or collar bone region, you tend to be too high on the chest and fail get the optimum results for your time and effort. The same holds true if the weights are too low, allowing them to drift too far down over the stomach area, thus working more shoulder than the chest.

  The best results can be attained by imagining a piece of string hanging down from your hand grip overhead, touching down like a pointer on your chest. You want that string or imaginary line to be on, or slightly below the nipple area, (about the width of your hand), whichever gives you the optimum effect. Refer back to the photo illustration in chapter 9.

- With the possible exception of rotating the wrists inward as suggested earlier, it is important to keep the position of the dumbbells the same throughout the entire repetition. If you get into the habit of overly turning, twisting, or changing the angle of the wrist during the exercise movement, you will have a tendency to affect more of the shoulder area than the pecs. That's not what we are after at this time.

  For the most part, keep the dumbbells in the same *parallel position to the ground* throughout the entire movement, from start to finish.

- Do not allow the shoulders at any time to *rotate forward* at the fully lowered position. This could injure your shoulder joint as well as delay your progress. Maintain strict form throughout.

- The negative resistance of the lowering phase can play just as important a role as in the upward phase IF you use it right. This is achieved by strictly controlling the ease in which you lower the weights on each rep, thus maintaining constant tension on the pecs throughout. Again, **you** control the descent, not gravity. This is most desirable for quick, efficient gains.

- Again, re-check the amount of weight. If you break form before you reach the minimum required number of reps per set, you have too much on.

  On the other hand, if you are cranking out more than 15 or 20 reps per set, you will need to add.

- Think in terms of "blowing the weights up" to aid you in proper breathing technique.

- Later on, this exercise may require further adaptation in technique on your part in order to achieve optimum results. As you become more experienced in weight training, you will get to know your body better and how it will respond to different stimuli. Never be afraid to change things around and experiment.

- If all else has failed up to this point, you can now try adding a little more weight resistance to this exercise.

OVERHEAD PRESS

- Concentrate entirely on the deltoids doing the work, **not the arms.**

- Avoid bouncing, jerking, or use of unnecessary momentum. Initiate each rep smoothly, correctly, yet powerfully.

- Give yourself a good ol' burning FLEX at the top of each rep, at the point your arms become fully extended (yet, stopping just short of locking the elbows).

  But pay close attention to make sure that you are not flexing more with your arms (triceps), rather than targeting strictly the deltoids. You will be amazed at the difference it makes. Think about this and try it again.

- Maintain full range of motion throughout each repetition. That is, all the way up and all the way down.

  Avoid being one of those who cheat themselves by bringing the bar only part or halfway down. This becomes common when attempting more weight than one is capable of doing correctly, and it shows!

- Avoid resting too long on either the top or bottom end of each rep. You should pause only for a short one count while flexing at the top, and then back down again. Keep it moving and I know you will be surprised.

- If you still have problems feeling what you think you should, try varying your hand grip on the bar by widening or narrowing your hands ever so slightly. It doesn't require much, only a couple inches at a time.

  Again, use a slightly relaxed grip with the weight resting on the bottom part or "heel" of the hand.

- Maintain a consistent area where the bar *lightly* touches (but not completely resting), during the bottom part of each rep. Often, as one fatigues, the technique worsens, such as the head beginning to drop or the bar stopping fairly short of starting position, (coming only half-way down).

  Double check the photo illustration on where it should be, then hit that same spot each and every time.

- Be true to yourself in using the correct amount of weight resistance. Add or subtract accordingly.

- Maintain correct body positioning. Make sure you keep yourself solid with back straight and feet flat on the floor. If not, you can expect diminishing results, possibly injury.

- Remember to use proper breathing technique. Exhale when pushing the bar overhead and inhale on the way down.

- If all else has failed up to this point, you can now try adding a little more weight resistance to this exercise.

<u>TRICEP EXTENSION</u>
(Standing)

- CONCENTRATE! Mentally isolate the tricep only. The forearm should be the one and only thing that moves.

- DO NOT allow the shoulders to sag, shrug or rotate. Keep them back and square, with the chest out.

- The position in which you are able to maintain the elbows is another important key to the effectiveness of this exercise.

  They MUST remain at your side, in one spot at all times, disallowing any unnecessary shifting from either the front or to the rear. They should act as a set pivot point from which all motion *revolves <u>around</u>*.

- *Be sure to FLEX during the very end of the extension phase*, the point at which most contraction occurs.

  If done correctly, you will almost immediately feel a burning sensation in the backs of your arms, with results soon to follow.

- It may be possible to achieve an even fuller stretch and better isolation, by *slightly* FLEXING the bicep during each rep, (at the up and starting position).

  This ensures you begin each rep from ground zero. That means a complete and dead stop, in hopes of avoiding any kind of help from unnecessary momentum.

- If you still have problems maintaining a perfect circular motion, try *thinking* of extending OUT front first, then DOWN. (But keep those elbows pinned to one spot.) This will truly aid you in getting the most out of this movement.

- The three muscles of the tricep can be stimulated in other distinct ways, but without changing exercises.

  Experiment by varying the distance of your hand spacing on the bar. Doing this will effect each muscle a little differently.

  An alternative would be to start the first set with hands together, then gradually work out wider as you begin sets 2 through 5.

- This time, try keeping your wrists firm and not let them sag backwards. Instead, try to get to the point where you can perform the entire motion with them curled forward and down. This will put a direct stimulation on the targeted area.

- Again, it should only be the triceps responsible for maintaining control throughout the upward return movement during each rep, rather than leaving it all up to gravity.

  Always remain in control of ALL motion.

- If all else fails, drop the weight a little. It can make all the difference.

- Avoid over-leaning or bending over too far during exercise. A *slight* inward lean is all there should be, no more.

  Having to cheat in this manner is another indication of using more weight than you can handle correctly.

- Proper breathing technique dictates you should exhale during the extension phase and inhale during the return.

- If all else has failed up to this point, you can now try adding a little more weight resistance to this exercise.

TRICEP EXTENSION
(on a bench)

The troubleshooting procedure here is basically the same as the previous standing tricep exercise earlier, except for these few additional ones listed.

- Make sure you keep your elbows solid. DO NOT at any time allow them to drift either to the front or to the back. This is not a pull-over exercise, as they must remain as stationary as possible.

- Check to see if you are keeping the elbows pointed inward and parallel to each other (not outward).

- Finish each rep with the bar directly over the head, *not the chest.* Think of it as a more over-centered position.

  Although this makes it more difficult, this technique ensures you maintain proper stimulation and further isolation of the tricep region.

- You must FLEX at the top of each rep and feel a full stretch while at the bottom.

- If available, substitute the straight bar for a specialized curl bar. This simple, but highly effect piece of hardware greatly enhances the effects of this exercise. Try it with either a narrow OR wide grip.

- Exhale as you extend upward and inhale as the bar is lowered.

- If all else has failed up to this point, you can now try adding a little more weight resistance to this exercise.

BENT-OVER ROWING

- First and foremost, ask yourself if you are **concentrating** only on the lat muscle itself. If not, get the brain into it.

- If you find concentrating difficult, many times it is because you feel the arms doing most of the work, particularly the biceps. Granted, although the emphasis is placed on the muscles of the back, there is no way to totally isolate it and not feel it in the arms at the same time.

  Instead, try to focus your thoughts into believing the hands and forearms are just *levers* or *hooks*, linking the bar to the shoulders. Convince yourself these attachments are powerless by themselves, unless you initiate and control all movement **beginning with the elbows**, on up through the muscles in the back.

  In short, create a mental image that blanks out any conscience feeling below the elbows.

- Try performing your repetitions extra slow on both the up and downward movements. Much slower than the other exercises.

  Sometimes this is what it finally takes to actually recruit as many of the back muscles as possible during this often stubborn, hard-to-isolate exercise. (Here, you may again have to decrease the weight a little more in order to be able to do it right.)

- In a loose fashion, try gripping the bar only with the fingers. Move the thumbs <u>from around the bar</u> and place them on top, next to the fingers.

- DO NOT jerk, or rear up, using the lower back in an attempt to initiate momentum. You not only delay results, but increase your chance of lower back injury.

  By having to cheat in this manner indicates that you are probably using too heavy a resistance in the first place. Continue to reduce the amount of weight until you are able to do each repetition SMOOTHLY and COMPLETELY, from a dead start to finish. Even if you have to resort to using an empty bar or broom handle, do it!

  You will instantly be amazed at what you will feel and the ease in which your technique will improve.

- Lower the bar in a SLOW and controlled manner each and every time. The negative aspect of this movement plays just as important a role as in the lifting phase.

- If you are still having problems, you should find that this next helpful hint should do the trick.

  The key in this exercise and most others that deal with the back, is in the positioning of the ELBOWS. If you only try one of these troubleshooting guides, let it be this one.

  THE ELBOWS <u>MUST</u>:

  Remain close to your side throughout the entire movement. Keep them pointed IN and UP, allowing them to lightly brush your sides.

  Last, but most importantly, you must LEAD with the elbows, moving them as far back BEHIND YOU as possible, each and every time you pull the bar up to touch the hip area.

- FLEX the lat muscles at the same time the elbows are fully up and behind you. A good way to do this is to hold each top position for a short one count.

- The arms and shoulders must **fully** relax at the bottom end of each rep, allowing more for a dead hang and a fully stretched position. This will ensure you start each rep from scratch, thus creating the utmost response possible from the lat muscles themselves.

- Another way to ensure a start-from-scratch bent over row, is to try *rolling* or *rotating* the shoulders forward and down at the bottom end of each rep, then pull upward.

  Again, if this particular alteration seems to do the trick, make sure you consistently enforce it on each and every rep of each and every set.

- Always check yourself to make sure you are maintaining solid form. It becomes easy to misjudge the angle of your body, bringing with it a tendency to raise up too high.

  Keep the back parallel or just above parallel to the floor, and avoid allowing the back to slouch or stoop, creating too much of an arch.

- What was just expressed in the previous suggestion may not hold true for everyone who tries it. I am referring to the correct angle of where the upper body should be throughout this exercise.

  Experiment further, if you must, by either raising or lowering the angle of your upper body, until maximum stimulation of the lats can be reached. You will know it when it happens.

Many have found the angle slightly higher than 90 degrees to be most beneficial (with this type of closed-grip technique only).

With the wider grips, others find that by bending way over until the head is even with the knees and using a little lighter resistance to be the ticket (those with no back problems). If you feel you can, give these a try.

- **Begin** and **end** each repetition from a dead stop. Do not swing the bar up. Again, re-check the amount of weight you are using.

- Do not over-grip! This will divert attention away from the lats, and more to the arms. The hands should be as relaxed as possible, yet, *just tight enough* to maintain adequate grip on the bar.

- If your knees are in the proper slightly-bent position, try pulling the bar up until your hands are *just over* the knees, then continue the upward movement by slightly brushing against the thighs for the rest of the way up, all the way until your hands touch the hip bones in the finished position.

  This will maintain a good rowing motion for adequate lat stimulation, rather than feeling it so much in the biceps.

- Instead of using a straight bar, try the exact same exercise with a curling bar or "T-bar" apparatus, if available. The specialized design makes for better hand placement along with providing a fuller range of motion.

- (Traditional Wide-grip technique) - After a certain period of time, it's possible you may experience some diminishing results. If this is the case, try varying your hand grip AND the area in which the bar touches, but keep all other thought patterns and motion technique the same.

  For example, try using an extra wide hand grip position, (wider than shoulder-width) only this time, pull the bar up each time into the midsection. This will tend to include more of the center back while increasing lower back density.

  This type of variation will give you a renewed feeling of stimulation into this exercise, while still working the necessary full range of lat and back muscles.

- In addition to a wider hand spacing, some find that by reversing their grip with palms facing outward, to provide yet another change-up effect to this exercise. (However, it does put a greater emphasis and dependency upon the biceps as a result.)

- You should exhale during the lifting phase and inhale while lowering.

- Finally, I believe the importance of the earlier suggestions bear repeating.

  LEAD WITH THE <u>ELBOWS</u> ON EACH REPETITION, MAKING SURE THEY ALWAYS TRAVEL AS FAR <u>BACK</u> AND <u>BEHIND</u> YOU AS POSSIBLE.

LAT PULL-DOWN

- *Concentrate*! You should be able to feel a full and complete stretch of the lat muscles in the area below and to the side of the armpit. Now, *think* those muscles into action. Do your best to allow only them to respond.

- Start and stop from a complete stretched position. By doing this on each rep ensures you much greater stimulation to a larger portion of the back than you would otherwise.

- As in the Bent-Over Rows, the most important thing here is the ELBOWS. Check yourself on each of the following steps;

    1) Focus on LEADING with the elbows.

    2) Keep them IN and close to your side *throughout the entire motion.*

    3) Last, but most importantly, the more you are able to move the elbows back behind you, the better the results will be.

- Experiment with various widths of hand grips, ranging from narrow to somewhat wider.

- For additional variation, use an extra wide grip and try pulling the bar down behind the head, at the same time, always making sure the bar touches the *lower* neck and shoulder area (not just the back of the head). This is often recognized as the more popular and traditional style.

- Use the same extra wide grip, only this time, pull the bar down in front and across the chest area. Double check the elbows. Here, they should point out to the side and still travel as far back behind you as possible. This will directly stimulate the upper most part of the lat muscle.

- Do not over-grip! Hold just tight enough to get the job done. If you have to, move the thumbs <u>from around the bar</u>, and place them on top next to the fingers.

- Remember to utilize the mind. Convince yourself into thinking that the hands are merely attachments or hooks connecting you to the bar. All conscience feelings from the elbows outward should be blanked out. Pull as much as you can with the upper back, not with the biceps.

    Putting yourself in this frame of thought will further aid you in isolating only the lat muscles.

- Do not jerk or hang on the bar in the desperate attempt to seek help in pulling it down.

  This should be a good indication that you have on too much resistance, therefore, you should continue to take weight off until you are able to execute only SMOOTH and COMPLETE repetitions.

- You should exhale as you pull down during the exertion phase, and inhale as you extend back to a full stretch.

- I believe the importance of the earlier suggestions bear repeating.

  LEAD WITH THE <u>ELBOWS</u> ON EACH REPETITION, MAKING SURE THEY ALWAYS TRAVEL AS FAR <u>BACK</u> AND <u>BEHIND</u> YOU AS POSSIBLE.

- If all else has failed up to this point, you can now try adding a little more weight resistance to this exercise.

INCLINE CURL

- This could possibly be one of the easier exercises to connect the mind with the muscle group you are working.

  Remember, you are *curling* the weight, not pulling, jerking, or swinging.

  Concentrate! Look down at the bicep, isolate it, force it to respond, watch it work, and watch it grow!

- If you still have trouble feeling what you think you should, have *patience*. If you felt little on the first set, YOU WILL feel it on the second set, third, and so on.

  Many times it is because most of the concentrated effort during the first set is used up in learning the exercise motion itself. Naturally, this takes time.

  Hang in there and don't give up. It will all come together with time and practice.

- If you are concentrating and yet still feel nothing, these next two troubleshooting ideas should do the trick.

    1) THE ELBOWS MUST NOT MOVE. They should be thought of only as a hinge that is nailed to one spot against to your side. Avoid allowing them to drift forward during the curling motion. If they move out of position, even just a little, the results will be drastically impaired. The only thing that should move are the forearms.

    2) YOU MUST FLEX AT BOTH ENDS. FLEX the biceps at the top position, while, just as importantly, *lightly* FLEXING the triceps in the extended position. This slight flexing of the triceps at the bottom actually helps relax and fully STRETCH the bicep, ensuring the entire bicep muscle is being worked through it's fullest range of motion. Try it and be amazed!

- While keeping the elbows in a set position, THINK or VISUALIZE curling the dumbbells up in a frontal circular motion (a full half circle), powered ONLY by the biceps. So long as the elbows DO NOT move, isolation should not be a problem.

- If you feel it more in the shoulders, particularly the frontal deltoid, this usually indicates you are either moving the elbows out of position, have too much weight on, or both. Re-check your weight.

- I'll say it again, this exercise requires nothing but strict isolation, which, unfortunately, makes it very easy for the inexperienced as well as some of the experienced to begin with too much weight.

Evaluate yourself honestly and ignore how much the person next to you is doing. *Take it off* and REALLY FEEL IT!

- Watch and make sure the dumbbells do not venture out away from the sides during the upward curling motion.

  Instead, curl the dumbbells up as close to your side as possible, even to the point where they lightly brush against the thighs each time they go by.

  Do the exact same thing during the downward movement as well.

- Watch your wrists during the curling motion. If they are twisting ever so slightly at the top end you are probably not getting everything this exercise has to offer.

  During the bottom end, at the time the dumbbells are in the hanging position, visualize curling the dumbbells as you would if you were curling a straight bar throughout the *entire* motion, especially when you reach the very top end. At that point, double-check the positioning of your wrists. Could you still visualize a straight bar across your chest? Or have the wrists twisted outward? Check yourself!

- If all else fails, simply decrease the angle of the backrest a little more by lowering it one notch.

- Exhale during the upward curl and inhale as the dumbbells are lowered. Remember to think of blowing the weights up.

- Later on, ONLY after having tried the earlier techniques for a considerable time, turn your wrists slightly inward *towards the thighs* on each upward curling movement. This should shift the elbows ever so slightly outward yet still retain solid form throughout.

- Experiment further by gradually rotating the wrists outward *throughout* and *during* the entire lift. This is when the palms of the hands begin from a natural inward hang at the bottom, while finishing at the top, facing up.

  These special adaptations of exercise will further stimulate the bicep in ways much different than you may have become used to.

- Try using the "hammer curl" technique. This is done by grasping the dumbbells like you would use a hammer. The dumbbells remain in a parallel position throughout the entire motion. Here, you should really feel it on the outside of the bicep.

- If you reach a point where you think you want more, go for the burn. Push yourself beyond the pain barrier, feeling as if the bicep is about to explode. By going this one extra step, you will notice a new peak to your bicep almost instantly.

- If all else has failed up to this point, you can now try adding a little more weight resistance to this exercise.

<u>BENT-KNEE SIT-UP</u>

- Isolation and concentration of the abdominal muscles are a must. Paint yourself a mental picture of the abdominal muscles forming during each and every motion. And I mean every repetition. Not once-in-a-while, not every other one, but each rep.

  Likewise, you will find that the better you are able to mentally control each movement, the better your exercise form and technique will also improve, thus reducing the chance of injury. Using this method of brain and body WILL make for speedy results.

- Picture yourself much like a tightly rolled newspaper. Tightly **roll** yourself to the up position, while just as importantly **unrolling** the abdominal muscles back to the down position. Always stay in control and be aware of just what is and is not doing the work.

- Try to keep the neck as relaxed as possible.

- Really FLEX the abs when crossing over and touching the opposite knee.

- If you so desire, go one step further and put a little more side twist into it, by re-focusing your line of sight straight **out to the side**, instead of always down at the opposite knee in front of you.

- Aim at keeping the arms pointed straight out to the side throughout, rather than pointed forward in a head-cradling fashion.

- To just touch the top of the knee may not be enough for some. Twist far enough so that your elbow aggressively touches the **outside** of the opposite knee. You should now feel the abs contract and FLEX without having to even think about it.

- Check to make sure you are travelling the full range of motion each time.

  All the way up..FLEX..then all the way down, until the fingers behind the head *lightly* touch the bench or floor, then back up again without resting. (Do not fully rest or relax at the bottom when stretched out, but rather strive to maintain a certain amount of abdominal tension throughout).

  This method of execution will stimulate AND bind together the full range of your midsection to the lower torso, starting from down in the groin area all the way up to the rib cage.

- Be aware of allowing the hip flexors to do most of the work. (Those frontal muscles in the hip that help lift the legs and initiate the sit up exercise.)

  Granted, they are an important part of this particular synchronization of muscles, but not what we are after. Do your best to keep them from over-dominating the work we are targeting for the abs. It all falls back on concentrating properly.

- When you begin to feel a strain in the neck, or begin to jerk and pull yourself up by the arms, it is here you should stop. You've reached your limit for that particular set.

  At this point you achieve little by breaking form and pushing on, except further increasing the chance of lower back injury.

- If you find yourself having trouble concentrating because you continue to pull or jerk yourself up by the arms, try this;

  Place your fingertips on the temples to the side of your head, instead of locking the hands behind the head. Keep them there throughout the entire exercise.

- If you eventually reach a point where little is being gained, raise the sit-up board one setting. As time goes by, continue to raise one setting at a time whenever you reach a point of feeling stagnate.

  However, do not change positions of the board too quickly. Concentrate and give each different setting an equal amount of trial and error as the one before. This should all happen over a considerable period of time, usually several months to years depending on the individual.

- If you eventually work up to being one of the rare few who find the highest setting of the board to be less and less a challenge, simply return it back to the floor and start all over again.

  You will be amazed at the renewed feeling you will get by starting over, even though it obviously appears easier.

- At this particular point, this far into the Troubleshooting suggestions, is the time I would say to go ahead and experiment on your own with different variations of exercise regarding the ab muscles. At this point, you should be fairly well experienced enough to know what works and what doesn't.

  But remember, when it comes to abdominal exercises, if you find it fairly easy to do, you are probably not getting as much out of it as you would like. Usually, the more difficult and isolated, the more productive.

- You shouldn't have a problem with your breathing technique during this exercise. It seems to come fairly natural, that is, exhaling on the upward phase and inhale on the downward phase.

AB-CROSS BURNOUT

- Strict isolation of the abdominal muscles is critical, and a rep should not be considered good just because you succeed in touching the knee. The mind-to-body thought process must go along with it. Keep working on it.

- YOUR ELBOWS MUST TOUCH THOSE KNEES, EACH AND EVERY TIME! Making sure you touch the knee is just as important as the thinking process. You must *DRIVE* the knee as far up the chest as possible on each rep. This seems to tie everything together and ensure you a tight, stimulated feeling every time.

- Avoid trying to elevate your upper body too high off the floor. Remember, this is not a sit-up. Here, only the shoulders and upper back lift slightly off the ground.

  Trying to come up too high each time creates an overly awkward feeling while increasing the chance for lower back injury.

- When bringing the knee up, keep it tightly tucked and *in line with your body*, disallowing it to travel too far out to the side. Some of which will depend upon flexibility.

- You must twist and FLEX at the top of each rep. If you have to, hold each top end position for a short one count. (The point at which the elbow touches the knee.)

- Synchronize yourself so that the locked fingers behind your head *lightly* touch the floor at the same time the heels of both feet do, thus ensuring a fuller stretch and fuller range of motion.

- Keep constant tension on the abs at all times, especially when hitting the stretched position. You can do this by allowing only the heels of your feet to lightly touch the floor, not the calves or back of the thighs.

  In short, never allow the legs to completely relax flat on the floor.

- Check to make sure your clasped hands remain <u>behind</u> the head rather than on top, especially after fatigue sets in.

  By allowing them to shift out of position, even if it's just a little, could reduce the amount of stimulation possible, thereby delaying results.

- Although the motion of this exercise appears to be relatively easy, it also can become quite inconsistent. At times, one can go through the motions and still not feel anything productive. If this is the case and you feel as though you've hit a dead end, try this next method ONLY if you have seriously tried the earlier suggestions.

Pick three visual points of reference at each body position.

(Body Position)

When you are in the flat, stretched out position, pick a consistent point or object **directly** above you, such as a light fixture or speck on the ceiling. This is the point you will directly focus on for that brief moment every time the back of your head touches the floor.

Next, pick out a point of reference on both extreme right and left sides in the same manner. Make sure each focal point is **directly** out to the side far enough to ensure an adequate twist at the top of each rep. Otherwise it becomes too easy to look down at the floor in front of you.

(Working Example)

While laying flat you focus on a <u>crack</u> in the ceiling, as you raise and twist to your left, your eyes pinpoint a <u>picture</u> on the wall, then back down again. The instant the back of your head lightly touches the floor on the return motion, you should again catch a glimpse of that same <u>crack</u> overhead, then raise up and twist to the right eyeballing <u>an electrical outlet</u> on the opposite wall. Simply repeat over and over until you finish the set.

Each reference point must be locked on and targeted, on each and every repetition. (This particular method should be done slowly to avoid possible dizziness.)

- When you begin to notice a straining of the neck muscles or find yourself jerking or pulling yourself up with the arms, you have probably reached total abdominal fatigue.

  It is best to stop at this point in the set, for once you begin to break form, no matter how many more you force yourself into doing, little is gained.

- Proper breathing technique usually takes care of itself. You should exhale when curling up and inhale deeply when lowering back to the stretched position.

- Above all, keep it simple. If you try one or all of the suggestions above, but find you are more confused than before, clear your mind and go back to the basics. In other words, get down on the floor and just do it!

Sometimes, thinking too much will hinder rather than help.

THE SQUAT

- Concentrate so that ONLY the thighs are doing the work. The key to isolation here, is to push off with the **heels** of your feet. Whether standing flat-footed or on a 2 X 4, keep the weight back on the heels while pushing up.

- Keep most of the weight centered over the heels on the *downward* movement as well. CONTROL is the big thing here, always moving slow and low.

- Remember to maintain constant tension on the quads throughout the entire set. This will further isolate and develop cuts and definition.

  But be careful not to go so far that you hyper-extend the knee joint into a locked position, especially when using any amount of weight. Reckless locking of the knees in this manner WILL lead to serious injury.

- You will find that if you think about constantly pushing the heels **into the floor**, you will be able to maintain constant tension and isolation on the quads. Of course, it all depends upon how well you can keep your balance.

- I will say it again, you must keep the <u>head up</u> and <u>back locked</u>. Allowing the head to drop or sporting a droopy back will undoubtedly hinder your overall center of gravity, thus greatly effecting the outcome of your efforts.

  Also, never underestimate the increased risk of spinal injury. Always keep the back tight and solid while keeping the head up!

- Try changing things around a little by experimenting with different foot placements.

  If you move them closer together, while at the same time keeping the knees together and directly out in front of you, you will notice a slight more stimulation of the outer quads. You may or may not be able to actually feel it at the time, but rest assured, the outer quad region is being reached in this manner. (Be sure to keep feet parallel to each other with toes pointed forward.)

  Inversely, by widening the legs and pointing the toes slightly out to the side, you will tend to stimulate more of the inner quads.

- Do not allow the legs to splay out too far to the sides when squatting. This will add undue stress to the knee joint while creating an unnatural range of movement. Keep the knees pointed in a forward direction throughout.

- EXPLODE upward on each and every rep.

  For those athletes in prime condition and carrying loftier goals, train the leg muscles to respond with dynamic explosiveness. Legs not only need to be strong, but functionally responsive as well. Just look at some of our superstar athletes we have today.

  But remember, <u>never bounce off the bottom</u>! Instead, lower yourself slowly on each rep until you reach the bottom, then carefully make sure you have pushed up a few inches FIRST, before finally ramming your way up. This will help prevent straining or tearing of the muscles and ligaments around the knees.

- Eventually, you should strive to get to the point you can squat without blocks or a 2 X 4 under your heels. It will take time, but in the long run, it will help maintain proper flexibility and balance overall.

- If you lack flexibility throughout the back of the leg, add calf, hamstring, and Achilles' tendon stretching exercises to your warm-up and stretching routine.

- After a considerable amount of time and experience, the addition of the Frontal Squat exercise seems to add more to the amount of thigh stimulation possible, from what you have eventually become accustomed. However, it is an exercise variation that may take some getting used to.

  Instead of behind the neck, the bar is positioned in front, high across the collar bone, resting on top of the shoulders with the forearms crossed at the wrist for additional support. Here, less weight than normal is used.

  This particular deviation from the normal Squat will require an increase in balance and upper body strength, but as you will soon find, the change is usually very productive. Again, it is usually restricted more for the athletically inclined.

- If all else has failed up to this point, you can now try adding a little more weight resistance to this exercise.

LEG EXTENSION

- Your concentrated effort should be on the isolation of the thigh muscles on both the upward AND downward movement. Look down and watch them work, *watch them develop.*

- Don't forget, give your legs a good FLEX when in the fully extended position.

  To ensure a good flex, some find that by holding the top part of each rep for a short one count really makes the difference.

- Check to be sure you are going the full range of motion and not just part or half way. Always go all the way up, and all the way down.

- If you find yourself beginning each lift by raising your buttocks of the bench, you probably have on too much resistance. Take it off!

  The beginning and end of each rep should be smooth and technically perfect.

- Keep it moving! DO NOT allow yourself to rest each time the weights touch the bottom of the rack. I repeat, the weights touch only slightly and for an instant, then back up you go again.

- Always try to maintain constant tension on the quad muscles throughout the entire exercise. This keeps you from banging the weights, prevents jerking of the knee, and quite simply, gets more out of the exercise overall.

- Try keeping the toes pointed either up or down during the entire movement, whichever provides the optimum effect.

  Usually, the toes-down technique does the best job in strictly targeting the thighs, whereas, when the toes are pointed up, the effects are spread out more evenly with the additional stretching of the calves and hamstrings.

- If you want to zero in on a more specific area of the quadriceps you can do so by simply moving the position of the knees.

  Exercising with the knees together will stimulate more of the middle and outside of the thigh, while widening them tends to stimulate more of the inner regions.

- Remember to blow the weights up. Exhale on the upward push and inhale deeply on the return stroke.

- If all else has failed up to this point, you can now try adding a little more weight resistance to this exercise.

LEG CURL

- Concentrate! Isolate only the hamstring muscles doing the work. Keep working on that mind/body link.

- Make sure you are doing this exercise in a half circle motion, a strict *curling* movement where the feet *rotate around* the set pivot points (your knees).

- KEEP THE BUTTOCKS DOWN. Do not allow it at any time to rise up. Instead, make the heels of your feet come up and touch your buttocks, not the other way around.

- If you have difficulty keeping the buttocks down, some find that by continually *pressing the hips and belly down onto the bench* throughout the entire motion, surprisingly, to have found a much more targeted, isolated effort overall. Granted, it makes the exercise harder to do, but also much more productive in the long run. Try it!

- FLEX the hamstrings at the top of every rep. Sometimes it helps to think of it as *pressing the heels into your buttocks* each time you hit the top position.

- As a bonus, go ahead and flex or squeeze the buttocks each time you hit the top end of every repetition. See what happens.

- Check to make sure you are executing each rep through its fullest range of motion. All the way up and all the way down. No shortcuts here either.

- Mentally AND physically be aware of the stretch feeling each time you *lower* your legs during the downward movement. In other words, just don't let gravity take over, YOU remain in control at all times.

- DO NOT rest between repetitions. Keep constant tension on the hamstrings during each and every repetition by only allowing the weights to *barely* touch at the bottom end, and only for an instant, before curling back up again.

  The timing and execution of the Leg Curl is much the same as in the Leg Extension exercise worked previously.

- If you continue to break form, such as jerking the weight up or arching the back, it probably means you have on too much weight. Take it off!

- You can slightly alter the effect on the hamstrings by experimenting with either the toes pointed straight out, or keeping them in a tucked position. Both work well, with personal feedback being the deciding factor.

- Proper breathing technique demands that you exhale on the upward curl, and inhale during the lowering phase.

- If all else has failed up to this point, you can now try adding a little more weight resistance to this exercise.

THE LUNGE

- One of the keys to the lunge, is to always strive to perfect your technique and motion of exercise. This then, should be more of a gliding movement rather than anything overly forceful.

  Here, you should learn to step out each time *SMOOTHLY*, while always maintaining constant muscle control.

- Eventually learn to develop a rhythm during this exercise. Just such an on-beat tempo often helps keep one more consistent throughout. If you have to, try it in front of a mirror for further visual help.

- If balance is a problem, you can replace the bar with light dumbbells in each hand hung down to your sides. All other technique should remain the same.

- It is very important to maintain the upper body's center of gravity by keeping the head up, shoulders square, and back locked. Avoid allowing the back to stoop or bend too far forward.

  Always check yourself in these areas.

- Mentally, force the *upper thigh* to initiate the upward push at the bottom, rather than beginning with any kind of a jerking or rocking motion. Keep it smooth, yet POWERFUL.

- **Concentrate** and feel the muscles of the quadriceps, groin and buttocks all work as one. Mentally isolate them from the rest of the body.

- Eventually learn to step out and land in a heel to toe fashion. In other words, the heel of the forward foot should land on the floor first, **before** coming to rest flat on the floor.

  Do the opposite for the way back up. Slightly rock the foot backwards, again, pushing off with the heel.

  In short, the heel should be the first thing to touch the floor on the way down, and the last thing to touch on the way up.

- Do not allow the forward knee to venture out to the side or too far out beyond the foot. Keep it in line with the body and pointed directly in out in front of you.

  This not only makes the movement more productive, but keeps the knee joint in a safer position.

- Want more? Try to reach as **full** a stretch as possible, by seeing to it that the knee of the trail leg stops slightly above, or just lightly touches the floor when **fully** extended behind you.

  This fully stretched position ensures those muscles of the buttocks, groin and hamstrings to be adequately stimulated, in turn, providing that all-important tighten and toning effect we all strive for. Here, you should really feel it.

- If you get to a point where you feel little is accomplished, add a **small** amount of weight to the bar resting across your neck and try it again. That should do it!

- Re-check your breathing technique. This is one of those movements that may feel awkward, creating the tendency to do just the opposite. You should inhale as you step out and exhale as you push yourself back up.

SQUAT EXPLOSION

- *Concentrate!* Begin each upward thrust with the *thighs*, nothing else.

- Keep it moving! There should be NO rest between repetitions.

- *Mentally* tie in to the LOWERING phase of coming back down to earth as well. This is very important.

  Disallow gravity to dictate the momentum of your descent, instead, YOU control it. The effects of learning such downward motion control will leave you amazed and productive.

- Learn to **sit back on your heels** during the lowering phase, in turn, forcing the thighs to constantly remain in control.

  This works especially well if the back remains in the same tightly locked, buttocks outward, position throughout (not just during the upward movement, but both up <u>and</u> down).

- If all else fails up to this point, don't overly concern yourself whether or not you are pushing off with the heels or the toes, just explode up naturally, allowing the leg muscles to work and react naturally as one. Here, thinking too much can be an unseen deterrent.

- FLEX your legs aggressively, immediately after your push off the floor.

- Teach yourself to land gracefully, coming down on the toes first, then with the rest of the foot, followed by bent knees for a soft, cushioned landing.

- Again, keep the back tightly arched (buttocks out) and the head up at all times. This will ensure you maintain proper balance and technique during the entire movement.

- Keep the knees pointed out in front of you at all times. Avoid getting into the habit of allowing them to splay outward. This will also help in maintaining a constant tension on the thigh area.

- Try to stay in the same area on the floor, landing exactly where you took off from. Avoid too much wandering around.

  The ability to remain in one spot throughout demonstrates good body control as well as increasing your chances of getting the most out of this exercise.

- DO NOT BOUNCE AT THE BOTTOM. Keep the up and down motion <u>smooth</u> <u>and fluid.</u>

  This is very important! Although it makes the effort a little more difficult, you will find not *nearly* as much is gained by *bouncing* off the bottom as you would by gently raising up a little first, BEFORE you initiate the upward thrust.

- Try varying your foot placement, either closer together or out a little wider than you first learned. This will stimulate your leg and groin muscles a little differently from what you have eventually become accustomed to.

  BUT, make sure your form stays solid (back tight and locked, head up, and knees pointed out in front, both when pushing up and when lowering back down).

- If after all is said and done and you feel as though you need just a little bit more, feel free to add a little weight to the bar. <u>That should do it!</u>

- For the athletically inclined, the mind-set here is to envision punching your head through the ceiling on each and every rep, again and again, until you can do no more. Train to Failure!

- Here again, breathing should take care of itself. Exhale when pushing up and inhale when lowering. Blow yourself upward!

LATERAL RAISE

- I'll say it again, and again, and again. Make sure you are continually concentrating on the muscle group you are working, if you can, even down to each individual muscle fiber.

- The angle of your wrist will play a surprising role in the successful development of your side and rear deltoids.

  Throughout the lifting phase, try rotating the wrist gradually downward so that the thumb points down and the little finger points up, as if you are pouring a pitcher of water.

- Always try to maintain position of the elbows during the lifting phase. They should remain in the same **slightly**-bent position throughout the entire exercise. Do not over-bend.

  Essentially, this should be a fairly straight arm movement.

- Avoid allowing the elbows to drop during the lifting phase. Keep them pointed **OUT** and **UP**.

- Pay close attention to keeping a wide circular motion *laterally*. The more fatigued you become throughout each set, the more difficult it becomes to maintain proper form.

  When this happens, try this method of thought; Think of lifting straight OUT to the side first, then UP. *Mentally* break it down into two steps. Lower them in the same fashion. Otherwise, it will remain too easy to allow the dumbbells to drift from the desired side pattern, over more to your front.

- Avoid shrugging or rotating the shoulders. Instead, keep the shoulders down and back, allowing them to pivot only at the shoulder joint. This will cut down on cheating.

- Do not swing the dumbbells to the up position. This can ONLY be acceptable when finishing out the last couple of reps in a *burn-out* situation. Otherwise, everything else should be flawless.

- Check to make sure you get the dumbbells all the way to the up position, *without shrugging* or breaking form, (not just half way).

- You should be FLEXING the deltoids at the top end of each repetition. This will ensure you get a good burn and speedy results.

- If you still have problems with your technique, re-check the amount of weight you are using. You probably have too much on.

   This is another one of those exercises that can be very deceptive in the amount of weight that is actually needed. Instead, start with a resistance you believe to be overly easy, even if it means resorting to using the smaller 2 1/2 or 5 pound single plates in each hand (due to the scarcity of a smaller pair of dumbbells). Try this and I know you will be surprised.

- This exercise is especially confusing when trying to develop proper breathing technique. Exhale during the lifting phase and inhale during the lowering phase.

   Watch it! It's easy to do just the opposite.

- Later, if you still want more, experiment further by switching to a bent-over stance. Bend forward until your upper body is parallel to the ground, some where around a 90 degree angle. Bend slightly at the knees while allowing the dumbbells to begin from a hanging position down by your feet. Now, use the same exercise technique as before. This particular variation directly stimulates the rear deltoid and upper back area.

- If all else has failed up to this point, you can now try adding a little more weight resistance to this exercise.

CALF RAISE

- Mentally isolate ONLY the combined effort of the calf muscles lifting you up, nothing else. In other words, the only parts doing the work should be from the knee down.

- Never begin by using a slight bounce or dip to initiate each upward movement, not at this time anyway. (Cheating in this manner is only acceptable at the very end of a set in an effort to complete a couple more than what would otherwise not be possible.)

- Don't forget to keep your thoughts focused on the downward movement as well, making sure you are not just *dropping* back down, but actually controlling the entire rate of return.

- Aggressively FLEX the calf muscles at the very top end of each repetition.

  Some experience an even greater effect by actually holding the top position for a short one count while flexing.

- If the concept of FLEXING fails to do the trick, try this;

  Each time, try to get up on the very *tip of your toes*, extending the _heels_ upward as high as possible, even to the point to where the knees bend forward a little.

  Here, the focus upon the *heel* works well most of the time.

- In keeping with the same line of thought as in the previous tip toe method, try popping the knees forward ever so slightly *and keep them there*, throughout the entire up and down movement. It makes for a more difficult exercise, but also more rewarding.

- If you are just a beginner and find it difficult in reaching at least 15 or more reps, restrict to using only your own body weight for resistance.

  If you still have problems using zero resistance, take heart, and keep trying. With further determination and patience, the extra reps WILL eventually come.

- For those a little more on the experienced side who just can't seem to reach those 25 or more *good* reps, reduce the amount of resistance. That's right. Swallow a little ego, then "Take it off" and really feel it.

- Keep it moving at the bottom end each time your heels touch the floor. Avoid any unnecessary rest delays.

To put it another way, as soon as the heels touch the floor and without bouncing, back up you go.

- Try varying your foot placement on the board by moving the feet either closer together or further apart.

- Along with varied foot placements, **foot direction** can also play an effective role in targeting specific calf muscle development.

  By pointing the toes inward, toward each other with the heels splayed out, one could expect to stimulate more of the outside of the calf, while reversing the direction, with heels together and toes pointing outward, the effect of stimulation tends to lean more to the inside of the calf.

- Although a little harder to do, try this; *Mentally* focus on pushing off with either the outside little toe of each foot, or the inside big toe, all dependent upon your main objective and feedback.

  Again, it is more the frame of thought we are looking for here, rather than actual physical capability of achieving such a feat.

- After a considerable amount of time of executing somewhat slow, deliberate repetitions, try pulling out all the stops and crank out as many reps you can in any one set, *as quickly as possible*. But again, just as long as technique remains strict.

  It's recommended you use less weight and high repetitions. Here, the burn won't be far behind.

- If you find one leg doing most of the work in comparison to the other, either you are not concentrating properly, or it could be because the calf of one leg is stronger than the other. This type of predicament is not all that uncommon, especially in beginners.

  In either case, even distribution of balance and strength will come to those who keep trying and never give up.

- If available, add to your arsenal of calf exercises by using any specialized calf machines some gyms and fitness clubs offer, such as; the standing or sitting calf raise machine, or various other designs similar in function.

  The standing version is much the same thing as in using a bar demonstrated earlier, however, it proves to be safer and much easier to use.

Likewise with the sitting apparatus. With knees tucked under pads in a secured fashion, this particular variation has the potential to bring a whole new dimension to the overall development of calf. If you find one, use it.

- Exhale as you rise up, inhale as you turn down.

- If all else has failed up to this point, you can now try adding a little more weight resistance to this exercise.

SIDE TWIST

- This is a good exercise to re-form that mind/body link toward a better waistline, an area many have lost touch with.

  Concentrate, isolate, mentally visualize, do what ever it takes in re-learning to open up and experience the renewed sensation of a strong, healthy, good looking midsection. Think It, Feel It, See It!

- Keep the stomach tense at all times. This will further help your mind to tie in and stay focused on the targeted area.

- Avoid using the arms to initiate movement. Instead, force only the abs to contract and pull the body around each time.

- Make sure you aggressively FLEX (tighten up or constrict) the entire range of stomach muscles, *each time the elbows come around in front of you.*

- In addition to flexing, try dipping the elbow slightly each time you hit the frontal position. This little trick will ensure you a complete and effective abdominal response.

- Maintain good posture. Head up and body straight.

- This is another one of those high rep exercises in which you try to do as many as you can, for however many sets you feel are necessary. I recommend at least 3 sets. When you get to the point of jerking or straining too hard in any one particular set, quit, you are then done for that set.

- Eventually, after a time when your range of motion and lower back flexibility have increased, make a point to draw a mental image of a vertical line separating the two equal halves of your body, centered directly in front of you. You then want the **elbow** (not just the hand) to cross or touch that particular imaginary point on each *full* twist. If necessary, watch yourself in a mirror, checking to make sure you are getting around far enough each time. (Refer back to the photo illustrations in chapter 10.)

  Also, allow the legs to float along with the twisting of your body. In other words, do not try too hard to hold them in a fixed position during the entire range of movement.

- Exhale each time you cross over. This outward forcing of air should occur naturally, much in part to the constricting of the stomach muscles themselves, in addition to the restricted body position.

BEGINNERS LAST CALL

It's no surprise to always find a few beginners who have given in to temptation by jumping head first into the more advanced, multi-set programs. Admirable, yes, but not very wise. Regardless, this is your choice so I will leave you this last hint of advice.

While undergoing multiple sets such as in the intermediate and advanced programs, you may feel as though you hit a brick wall during set #2, #3, and so on, in any one particular exercise leaving you unable to meet the minimum required number of repetitions (6). It is the point your body becomes weak and you're arms start to shake. Take heart, for this is quite normal.

Often one ponders how fatigue sets in so quickly after doing only one set. Again, this is probably because your muscles are not used to being pushed beyond their normal limits for such an extended time. Remember, this is all still new and very different.

In this situation, and only if you have to, go ahead and break the "M.E.T." concept rule established earlier in chapter seven called, "Keep It There!". In short, do what it takes in the beginning to make sure you are able to get at least six reps out of each set before trouble sets in, *even if it means taking off more weight before or after a troublesome set.* Take the Bench Press exercise for example, with the intention of performing a total of three sets.

On your first set you complete 12 or more reps and feel pretty good about it. On the second set you complete 7. You are still OK. But on the third set you are only able to complete 4 repetitions before reaching total muscle fatigue.

This brings you out of the minimum range of the required 6-12 number of reps for a set.

Therefore, you must decrease the amount of weight every time *before* you begin your third set on the Bench Press, until you are eventually able to accomplish at least 6 or more reps.

Eventually, your levels of strength and endurance will increase with time and effort, allowing you to maintain the same amount of resistance from the first set to the last, without having to subtract.

One more time, if you are unable to complete at least 6 good reps in any one set, you have added too much weight.

FOOD REFERENCE GUIDE

This food composition listing is to be used in conjunction with what is outlined earlier in chapter four, "Let's Eat."

However, you may notice something unusual about some of the foods listed with regard to their respective calorie and fat content. For example, one food may contain a hundred or more calories, but contain only a trace or zero amount of fat.

The major difference here is, *the source of where those calories came from,* instead of the obvious total number. In such cases, you shouldn't overly concern yourself with these types of foods, as long as the fat gram content remains low.

Of course, not every food or food combination is listed. This listing is only a reference guide to assist you in getting started, thus forcing you to eventually do your own food label computations. Find it! Figure it! Learn to live with it!

DESCRIPTION OF FOOD	AMOUNT PER SERVING	FAT (GRAMS)	FOOD ENERGY (CALORIES)
1000 ISLAND, SALAD DRSNG, LOCAL	1 TBSP	2	25
1000 ISLAND, SALAD DRSNG, REGLR	1 TBSP	6	60
100% NATURAL CEREAL	1 OZ	6	135
40% BRAN FLAKES, KELLOGG'S	1 OZ	1	90
40% BRAN FLAKES, POST	1 OZ	0	90
ALFALFA SEEDS, SPROUTED, RAW	1 CUP	0	10
ALL-BRAN CEREAL	1 OZ	1	70
ALMONDS, SLIVERED	1 CUP	70	795
ALMONDS, WHOLE	1 OZ	15	165
ANGELFOOD CAKE, FROM MIX	1 CAKE	2	1510
ANGELFOOD CAKE, FROM MIX	1 PIECE	0	125
APPLE JUICE, CANNED	1 CUP	0	115
APPLE PIE	1 PIE	105	2420
APPLE PIE	1 PIECE	18	405
APPLESAUCE, CANNED, SWEETENED	1 CUP	0	195

DESCRIPTION OF FOOD	AMOUNT PER SERVING	FAT (GRAMS)	FOOD ENERGY (CALORIES)
APPLESAUCE, CANNED, UNSWEETENED	1 CUP	0	105
APPLES, DRIED, SULFURED	10 RINGS	0	155
APPLES, RAW, PEELED, SLICED	1 CUP	0	65
APPLES, RAW, UNPEELED, 2 PER LB	1 APPLE	1	125
APPLES, RAW, UNPEELED, 3 PER LB	1 APPLE	0	80
APRICOT NECTAR, NO ADDED VIT C	1 CUP	0	140
APRICOTS, CANNED, JUICE PACK	1 CUP	0	120
APRICOTS, CANNED, JUICE PACK	3 HALVES	0	40
APRICOTS, DRIED, COOKED,UNSWTN	1 CUP	0	210
APRICOTS, DRIED, UNCOOKED	1 CUP	1	310
APRICOTS, RAW	3 APRCOT	0	50
APRICOT, CANNED, HEAVY SYRUP	1 CUP	0	215
APRICOT, CANNED, HEAVY SYRUP	3 HALVES	0	70
ARTICHOKES, GLOBE, COOKED, DRN	1 ARTCHK	0	55
ASPARAGUS, CKD FRM FRZ,DRN,CUT	1 CUP	1	50
ASPARAGUS, CKD FRM FRZ,DR,SPER	4 SPEARS	0	15
ASPARAGUS, CKD FRM RAW, DR,CUT	1 CUP	1	45
ASPARAGUS, CKD FRM RAW,DR,SPER	4 SPEARS	0	15
ASPARAGUS,CANNED, SPEARS,NOSALT	4 SPEARS	0	10
ASPARAGUS,CANNED, SPEARS, W/SALT	4 SPEARS	0	10
AVOCADOS, CALIFORNIA	1 AVOCDO	30	305
AVOCADOS, FLORIDA	1 AVOCDO	27	340
BAGELS, EGG	1 BAGEL	2	200
BAGELS, PLAIN	1 BAGEL	2	200
BAKING POWDER, LOW SODIUM	1 TSP	0	5
BAKING POWDER, STRGHT PHOSPHAT	1 TSP	0	5
BAKING POWDER, SAS, CA PO4	1 TSP	0	5
BAKING POWDER, SAS,CAPO4+CASO4	1 TSP	0	5
BAKING PWDR BISCUITS, FROM MIX	1 BISCUT	3	95
BAKING PWDR BISCUITS, HOMERECPE	1 BISCUT	5	100

Description of Food	Amount Per Serving	Fat (Grams)	Food Energy (Calories)
BAKING PWDR BISCUITS,REFRGDOGH	1 BISCUT	2	65
BAMBOO SHOOTS, CANNED, DRAINED	1 CUP	1	25
BANANAS	1 BANANA	1	105
BANANAS, SLICED	1 CUP	1	140
BARBECUE SAUCE	1 TBSP	0	10
BARLEY, PEARLED, LIGHT, UNCOOKD	1 CUP	2	700
BEAN SPROUTS, MUNG, COOKD,DRAN	1 CUP	0	25
BEAN SPROUTS, MUNG, RAW	1 CUP	0	3
BEAN WITH BACON SOUP, CANNED	1 CUP	6	170
BEANS,DRY,CANNED, W/FRANKFURTER	1 CUP	18	365
BEANS,DRY,CANNED, W/PORK+SWTSCE	1 CUP	12	385
BEANS,DRY,CANNED, W/PORK+TOMSCE	1 CUP	7	310
BEEF AND VEGETABLE STEW,HM RCP	1 CUP	11	220
BEEF BROTH, BOULLN, CONSM,CNND	1 CUP	1	15
BEEF GRAVY, CANNED	1 CUP	5	125
BEEF HEART, BRAISED	3 OZ	5	150
BEEF LIVER, FRIED	3 OZ	7	185
BEEF NOODLE SOUP, CANNED	1 CUP	3	85
BEEF POTPIE, HOME RECIPE	1 PIECE	30	515
BEEF ROAST, EYE O RND, LEAN	2.6 OZ	5	135
BEEF ROAST, EYE O RND, LEAN+FAT	3 OZ	12	205
BEEF ROAST, RIB, LEAN ONLY	2.2 OZ	9	150
BEEF ROAST, RIB, LEAN + FAT	3 OZ	26	315
BEEF STEAK,SIRLOIN, BROIL,LEAN	2.5 OZ	6	150
BEEF STEAK,SIRLOIN, BROIL,LN+FT	3 OZ	15	240
BEEF, CANNED, CORNED	3 OZ	10	185
BEEF, CKD,BTTM ROUND, LEAN ONLY	2.8 OZ	8	175
BEEF, CKD,BTTM ROUND, LEAN+ FAT	3 OZ	13	220
BEEF, CKD,CHUCK BLADE, LEANONLY	2.2 OZ	9	170
BEEF, CKD,CHUCK BLADE, LEAN+FAT	3 OZ	26	325

Description of Food	Amount Per Serving	Fat (Grams)	Food Energy (Calories)
BEEF, DRIED, CHIPPED	2.5 OZ	4	145
BEER, LIGHT	12 FL OZ	0	95
BEER, REGULAR	12 FL OZ	0	150
BEET GREENS, COOKED, DRAINED	1 CUP	0	40
BEETS, CANNED, DRAINED, NO SALT	1 CUP	0	55
BEETS, CANNED, DRAINED, W/ SALT	1 CUP	0	55
BEETS, COOKED, DRAINED, DICED	1 CUP	0	55
BEETS, COOKED, DRAINED, WHOLE	2 BEETS	0	30
BLACK-EYED PEAS, DRY, COOKED	1 CUP	1	190
BLACK BEANS, DRY, COOKED,DRAND	1 CUP	1	225
BLACKBERRIES, RAW	1 CUP	1	75
BLACKEYE PEAS, IMMATR, RAW,CKED	1 CUP	1	180
BLACKEYE PEAS,IMMTR, FRZN,CKED	1 CUP	1	225
BLUE CHEESE	1 OZ	8	100
BLUE CHEESE SALADDRESSING	1 TBSP	8	75
BLUEBERRIES, FROZEN, SWEETENED	1 CUP	0	185
BLUEBERRIES, FROZEN, SWEETENED	10 OZ	0	230
BLUEBERRIES, RAW	1 CUP	1	80
BLUEBERRY MUFFINS, HOME RECIPE	1 MUFFIN	5	135
BLUEBERRY MUFFINS, FROM COM MIX	1 MUFFIN	5	140
BLUEBERRY PIE	1 PIE	102	2285
BLUEBERRY PIE	1 PIECE	17	380
BOLOGNA	2 SLICES	16	180
BOSTON BROWN BREAD, W/WHTECRNM	1 SLICE	1	95
BOSTON BROWN BREAD,W/YLLWCRNML	1 SLICE	1	95
BOUILLON, DEHYDRTD,UNPREPARED	1 PKT	1	15
BRAN MUFFINS, FROM COMMERL MIX	1 MUFFIN	4	140
BRAN MUFFINS,HOME RECIPE	1 MUFFIN	6	125
BRAUNSCHWEIGER	2 SLICES	18	205
BRAZIL NUTS	1 OZ	19	185

Description of Food	Amount Per Serving	Fat (Grams)	Food Energy (Calories)
BREAD STUFFING,FROM MX,DRYTYPE	1 CUP	31	500
BREAD STUFFING,FROM MX,MOIST	1 CUP	26	420
BREADCRUMBS, DRY,GRATED	1 CUP	5	390
BROCCOLI, FRZN, COOKED,DRANED	1 CUP	0	50
BROCCOLI, FRZN, COOKED,DRANED	1 PIECE	0	10
BROCCOLI, RAW	1 SPEAR	1	40
BROCCOLI, RAW, COOKED,DRAINED	1 CUP	0	45
BROCCOLI, RAW, COOKED,DRAINED	1 SPEAR	1	50
BROWN AND SERVESAUSAGE,BRWND	1 LINK	5	50
BROWN GRAVY FROM DRY MIX	1 CUP	2	80
BROWNIES W/ NUTS, FRM HOME RECP	1 BROWNE	6	95
BROWNIES W/ NUTS,FRSTNG,CMMRCL	1 BROWNE	4	100
BRUSSELS SPROUTS, FRZN,COOKED	1 CUP	1	65
BRUSSELS SPROUTS,RAW, COOKED	1 CUP	1	60
BUCKWHEAT FLOUR,LIGHT, SIFTED	1 CUP	1	340
BULGUR, UNCOOKED	1 CUP	3	600
BUTTERMILK, DRIED	1 CUP	7	465
BUTTERMILK, FLUID	1 CUP	2	100
BUTTER, SALTED	1 PAT	4	35
BUTTER, SALTED	1 TBSP	11	100
BUTTER, SALTED	1/2 CUP	92	810
BUTTER, UNSALTED	1 PAT	4	35
BUTTER, UNSALTED	1 TBSP	11	100
BUTTER, UNSALTED	1/2 CUP	92	810
CABBAGE, CHINESE,PAK-CHOI,CKD	1 CUP	0	20
CABBAGE, CHINESE,PE-TSAI, RAW	1 CUP	0	10
CABBAGE, COMMON, COOKED, DRNED	1 CUP	0	30
CABBAGE, COMMON, RAW	1 CUP	0	15
CABBAGE, RED, RAW	1 CUP	0	20
CABBAGE, SAVOY, RAW	1 CUP	0	20

Description of Food	Amount Per Serving	Fat (Grams)	Food Energy (Calories)
CAKE OR PASTRY FLOUR, SIFTED	1 CUP	1	350
CAMEMBERT CHEESE	1 WEDGE	9	115
CANTALOUP, RAW	1/2 MELN	1	95
CAP'N CRUNCH CEREAL	1 OZ	3	120
CARAMELS, PLAIN ORCHOCOLATE	1 OZ	3	115
CAROB FLOUR	1 CUP	0	255
CARROT CAKE,CREMCHESEFRST,REC	1 CAKE	328	6175
CARROT CAKE,CREMCHESEFRST,REC	1 PIECE	21	385
CARROTS, CANNED, DRN,W/ SALT	1 CUP	0	35
CARROTS, CANNED,DRND,W/O SALT	1 CUP	0	35
CARROTS, COOKEDFROM FROZEN	1 CUP	0	55
CARROTS, COOKEDFROM RAW	1 CUP	0	70
CARROTS, RAW, GRATED	1 CUP	0	45
CARROTS, RAW, WHOLE	1 CARROT	0	30
CASHEW NUTS, DRY, ROASTD,SALTED	1 OZ	13	165
CASHEW NUTS, DRY, ROASTD,UNSALT	1 CUP	63	785
CASHEW NUTS, DRY, ROASTD,UNSALT	1 OZ	13	165
CASHEW NUTS, DRY ROASTED,SALTD	1 CUP	63	785
CASHEW NUTS, OIL ROASTD,SALTED	1 CUP	63	750
CASHEW NUTS, OIL ROASTD,SALTED	1 OZ	14	165
CASHEW NUTS, OIL ROASTD,UNSALT	1 CUP	63	750
CASHEW NUTS, OIL ROASTD,UNSALT	1 OZ	14	165
CATSUP	1 CUP	1	290
CATSUP	1 TBSP	0	15
CAULIFLOWER, COOKED FROM FROZN	1 CUP	0	35
CAULIFLOWER, COOKED FROM RAW	1 CUP	0	30
CAULIFLOWER, RAW	1 CUP	0	25
CELERY SEED	1 TSP	1	10
CELERY, PASCAL TYPE, RAW,PIECE	1 CUP	0	20
CELERY, PASCAL TYPE, RAW,STALK	1 STALK	0	5

Description of Food	Amount Per Serving	Fat (Grams)	Food Energy (Calories)
CHEDDAR CHEESE	1 CU IN	6	70
CHEDDAR CHEESE	1 OZ	9	115
CHEDDDAR CHEESE, SHREDDED	1 CUP	37	455
CHEERIOS CEREAL	1 OZ	2	110
CHEESE CRACKERS, PLAIN	10 CRACK	3	50
CHEESE CRACKERS,SANDWCH,PEANT	1 SANDWH	2	40
CHEESE SAUCEW/ MILK, FRM MIX	1 CUP	17	305
CHEESEBURGER, 4OZ PATTY	1 SANDWH	31	525
CHEESEBURGER, REGULAR	1 SANDWH	15	300
CHEESECAKE	1 CAKE	213	3350
CHEESECAKE	1 PIECE	18	280
CHERRIES, SOUR,RED,CANND,WATER	1 CUP	0	90
CHERRIES, SWEET, RAW	10 CHERY	1	50
CHERRY PIE	1 PIE	107	2465
CHERRY PIE	1 PIECE	18	410
CHESTNUTS, EUROPEAN, ROASTED	1 CUP	3	350
CHICKEN A LA KING,HOME RECIPE	1 CUP	34	470
CHICKEN AND NOODLES,HOME RECP	1 CUP	18	365
CHICKEN CHOW MEIN,CANNED	1 CUP	0	95
CHICKEN CHOW MEIN,HOME RECIPE	1 CUP	10	255
CHICKEN FRANKFURTER	1 FRANK	9	115
CHICKEN GRAVYFROM DRY MIX	1 CUP	2	85
CHICKEN GRAVY, CANNED	1 CUP	14	190
CHICKEN LIVER, COOKED	1 LIVER	1	30
CHICKEN NOODLE SOUP,CANNED	1 CUP	2	75
CHICKEN NOODLE SOUP,DEHYD,PRPD	1 PKT	1	40
CHICKEN POTPIE,HOME RECIPE	1 PIECE	31	545
CHICKEN RICE SOUP, CANNED	1 CUP	2	60
CHICKEN ROLL, LIGHT	2 SLICES	4	90
CHICKEN, CANNED,BONELESS	5 OZ	11	235

Description of Food	Amount Per Serving	Fat (Grams)	Food Energy (Calories)
CHICKEN, FRIED, BATTER,BREAST	4.9 OZ	18	365
CHICKEN, FRIED, BATTER,DRMSTCK	2.5 OZ	11	195
CHICKEN, FRIED, FLOUR,BREAST	3.5 OZ	9	220
CHICKEN, FRIED, FLOUR,DRMSTCK	1.7 OZ	7	120
CHICKEN, ROASTED, BREAST	3.0 OZ	3	140
CHICKEN, ROASTED,DRUMSTICK	1.6 OZ	2	75
CHICKEN, STEWED,LIGHT + DARK	1 CUP	9	250
CHICKPEAS, COOKED,DRAINED	1 CUP	4	270
CHILI CON CARNE W/ BEANS, CNND	1 CUP	16	340
CHILI POWDER	1 TSP	0	10
CHOCOLATE CHIP COOKIES,COMMRCL	4 COOKIE	9	180
CHOCOLATE CHIP COOKIES,HME RCP	4 COOKIE	11	185
CHOCOLATE CHIP COOKIES,REFRIG	4 COOKIE	11	225
CHOCOLATE MILK,LOWFAT 1%	1 CUP	3	160
CHOCOLATE MILK,LOWFAT 2%	1 CUP	5	180
CHOCOLATE MILK, REGULAR	1 CUP	8	210
CHOCOLATE, BITTER OT BAKING	1 OZ	15	145
CHOP SUEY W/ BEEF + PORK, HMRCP	1 CUP	17	300
CINNAMON	1 TSP	0	5
CLAM CHOWDER, MANHATTAN, CANND	1 CUP	2	80
CLAM CHOWDER, NEW ENG,W/ MILK	1 CUP	7	165
CLAMS, CANNED, DRAINED	3 OZ	2	85
CLAMS, RAW	3 OZ	1	65
CLUB SODA	12 FL OZ	0	0
COCA PWDR W/O NOFAT DRYMLK,PRD	1 SERVNG	9	225
COCA PWDR W/O NONFAT DRY MILK	3/4 OZ	1	75
COCOA PWDR WITH NONFAT DRYMILK	1 OZ	1	100
COCOA PWDR W/ NOFAT DRMLK,PRPD	1 SERVNG	1	100
COCONUT, DRIED, SWEETND,SHREDD	1 CUP	33	470
COCONUT, RAW, PIECE	1 PIECE	15	160

DESCRIPTION OF FOOD	AMOUNT PER SERVING	FAT (GRAMS)	FOOD ENERGY (CALORIES)
COCONUT, RAW, SHREDDED	1 CUP	27	285
COFFEECAKE, CRUMB, FROM MIX	1 CAKE	41	1385
COFFEECAKE, CRUMB, FROM MIX	1 PIECE	7	230
COFFEE, BREWED	6 FL OZ	0	0
COFFEE, INSTANT, PREPARED	6 FL OZ	0	0
COLA, DIET, ASPARTAME ONLY	12 FL OZ	0	0
COLA, DIET ASPRTAME + SACCHRN	12 FL OZ	0	0
COLA, DIET SACCHARIN ONLY	12 FL OZ	0	0
COLA, REGULAR	12 FL OZ	0	160
COLLARDS, COOKED FROM FROZEN	1 CUP	1	60
COLLARDS, COOKED FROM RAW	1 CUP	0	25
COOKED SALAD DRSSING HOME RCP	1 TBSP	2	25
CORN CHIPS	1 OZ	9	155
CORN FLAKES, KELLOGG'S	1 OZ	0	110
CORN FLAKES, TOASTIES	1 OZ	0	110
CORN GRITS, COOKED INSTANT	1 PKT	0	80
CORN GRITS,CKD,REG WHTE,NOSALT	1 CUP	0	145
CORN GRITS,CKD,REG WHTE,W/SALT	1 CUP	0	145
CORN GRITS,CKD,REG YLLW,NOSALT	1 CUP	0	145
CORN GRITS,CKD,REG YLLW,W/SALT	1 CUP	0	145
CORN MUFFINS, FROM COMMERL MIX	1 MUFFIN	6	145
CORN MUFFINS, HOME RECIPE	1 MUFFIN	5	145
CORN OIL	1 CUP	218	1925
CORN OIL	1 TBSP	14	125
CORNMEAL,BOLTED DRY FORM	1 CUP	4	440
CORNMEAL,DEGERMED ENRCHED,COOK	1 CUP	0	120
CORNMEAL,DEGERMED ENRICHED,DRY	1 CUP	2	500
CORNMEAL,WHOLE-GRND UNBOLT,DRY	1 CUP	5	435
CORN, CNND,CRM STL WHIT,NO SAL	1 CUP	1	185
CORN, CNND,CRM STL WHIT,W/SALT	1 CUP	1	185

281

DESCRIPTION OF FOOD	AMOUNT PER SERVING	FAT (GRAMS)	FOOD ENERGY (CALORIES)
CORN, CNND,CRM STL YLLW,NO SAL	1 CUP	1	185
CORN, CNND,CRM STL YLLW,W/SALT	1 CUP	1	185
CORN, COOKED FRM FROZN, WHITE	1 CUP	0	135
CORN, COOKED FRMFROZN, WHITE	1 EAR	0	60
CORN, COOKED FRMFROZN, YELLOW	1 CUP	0	135
CORN, COOKED FRM FROZN, YELLOW	1 EAR	0	60
CORN, COOKEDFROM RAW, WHITE	1 EAR	1	85
CORN, COOKEDFROM RAW, YELLOW	1 EAR	1	85
CORN,CNND,WHL KRNLWHTE,NO SAL	1 CUP	1	165
CORN,CNND,WHL KRNLWHTE,W/SALT	1 CUP	1	165
CORN,CNND,WHL KRNLYLLW,NO SAL	1 CUP	1	165
CORN,CNND,WHL KRNLYLLW,W/SALT	1 CUP	1	165
COTTAGE CHEESE,CREMD LRGE CURD	1 CUP	10	235
COTTAGE CHEESE,CREMD SMLL CURD	1 CUP	9	215
COTTAGE CHEESE,CREMD W/FRUIT	1 CUP	8	280
COTTAGE CHEESE LOWFAT 2%	1 CUP	4	205
COTTAGE CHEESE UNCREAMED	1 CUP	1	125
CR OF CHICKEN SOUP W/ H20,CNND	1 CUP	7	115
CR OF CHICKEN SOUP W/ MLK,CNND	1 CUP	11	190
CR OF MUSHROM SOUP W/ H2O,CNND	1 CUP	9	130
CR OF MUSHROM SOUPW/ MLK,CNND	1 CUP	14	205
CRABMEAT, CANNED	1 CUP	3	135
CRACKED-WHEAT BREAD	1 LOAF	16	1190
CRACKED-WHEAT BREAD	1 SLICE	1	65
CRACKED-WHEAT BREAD TOASTED	1 SLICE	1	65
CRANBERRY JUICE COCKTAL W/VITC	1 CUP	0	145
CRANBERRY SAUCE, CANNED SWTND	1 CUP	0	420
CREAM CHEESE	1 OZ	10	100
CREAM OF WHEAT,CKD MIX N EAT	1 PKT	0	100
CREME PIE	1 PIE	139	2710

DESCRIPTION OF FOOD	AMOUNT PER SERVING	FAT (GRAMS)	FOOD ENERGY (CALORIES)
CREME PIE	1 PIECE	23	455
CRM WHEAT,CKD, QUICK NO SALT	1 CUP	0	140
CRM WHEAT,CKD,QUICK W/ SALT	1 CUP	0	140
CRM WHEAT,CKD,REG,INST NO SALT	1 CUP	0	140
CRM WHEAT,CKD,REG,INST W/SALT	1 CUP	0	140
CROISSANTS	1 CROSST	12	235
CUCUMBER, W/ PEEL	6 SLICES	0	5
CURRY POWDER	1 TSP	0	5
CUSTARD PIE	1 PIE	101	1985
CUSTARD PIE	1 PIECE	17	330
CUSTARD, BAKED	1 CUP	15	305
DANDELION GREENS COOKED, DRND	1 CUP	1	35
DANISH PASTRY, FRUIT	1 PASTRY	13	235
DANISH PASTRY, PLAIN NO NUTS	1 OZ	6	110
DANISH PASTRY, PLAIN NO NUTS	1 PASTRY	12	220
DANISH PASTRY, PLAIN NO NUTS	1 RING	71	1305
DATES	10 DATES	0	230
DATES, CHOPPED	1 CUP	1	490
DEVIL'S FOOD CAKE CHOCFRST,FMX	1 CAKE	136	3755
DEVIL'S FOOD CAKE CHOCFRST,FMX	1 CUPCAK	4	120
DEVIL'S FOOD CAKE CHOCFRST,FMX	1 PIECE	8	235
DOUGHNUTS, CAKE TYPE PLAIN	1 DONUT	12	210
DOUGHNUTS, YEAST-LEAVEND, GLZED	1 DONUT	13	235
DUCK, ROASTEDFLESH ONLY	1/2 DUCK	25	445
EGGNOG	1 CUP	19	340
EGGPLANT, COOKED STEAMED	1 CUP	0	25
EGGS, COOKED	1 CUP	1	200
EVAPORATED MILK WHOLE, CANNED	1 CUP	19	340
FATS, COOKING/VEGETBL SHORTENG	1 CUP	205	1810
FATS, COOKING/VEGETBL SHORTENG	1 TBSP	13	115

DESCRIPTION OF FOOD	AMOUNT PER SERVING	FAT (GRAMS)	FOOD ENERGY (CALORIES)
FETA	1 OZ	6	75
FIG BARS	4 COOKIE	4	210
FIGS, DRIED	10 FIGS	2	475
FILBERTS, (HAZELNUTS) CHOPPED	1 CUP	72	725
FILBERTS, (HAZELNUTS) CHOPPED	1 OZ	18	180
FISH SANDWICH, LGE W/O CHEESE	1 SANDWH	27	470
FISH SANDWICH, REG W/ CHEESE	1 SANDWH	23	420
FISH STICKS, FROZEN REHEATED	1 STICK	3	70
FLOUNDER OR SOLEBAKED, BUTTR	3 OZ	6	120
FLOUNDER OR SOLE BAKED,MARGRN	3 OZ	6	120
FLOUNDER OR SOLE BAKED,W/OFAT	3 OZ	1	80
FONDANT, UNCOATED	1 OZ	0	105
FRANKFURTER, COOKED	1 FRANK	13	145
FRENCH BREAD	1 SLICE	1	100
FRENCH OR VIENNA BREAD	1 LOAF	18	1270
FRENCH SALAD DRESSINGLOCAL OR	1 TBSP	2	25
FRENCH SALAD DRESSING REGULAR	1 TBSP	9	85
FRENCH TOAST HOME RECIPE	1 SLICE	7	155
FRIED PIE, APPLE	1 PIE	14	255
FRIED PIE, CHERRY	1 PIE	14	250
FROOT LOOPS CEREAL	1 OZ	1	110
FRUIT COCKTAIL,CNND HEAVYSYRUP	1 CUP	0	185
FRUIT COCKTAIL,CNND JUICE PACK	1 CUP	0	115
FRUIT PUNCH DRINK CANNED	6 FL OZ	0	85
FRUITCAKE,DARK, FROM HOMERECIP	1 CAKE	228	5185
FRUITCAKE,DARK, FROM HOMERECIP	1 PIECE	7	165
FUDGE, CHOCOLATE, PLAIN	1 OZ	3	115
GARLIC POWDER	1 TSP	0	10
GELATIN DESSERT PREPARED	1/2 CUP	0	70
GELATIN, DRY	1 ENVELP	0	25

Description of Food	Amount Per Serving	Fat (Grams)	Food Energy (Calories)
GINGER ALE	12 FL OZ	0	125
GINGERBREAD CAKE FROM MIX	1 CAKE	39	1575
GINGERBREAD CAKE FROM MIX	1 PIECE	4	175
GIN,RUM,VODKA WHISKY 80-PROOF	1.5 F OZ	0	95
GIN,RUM,VODKA,WHISKY 86-PROOF	1.5 F OZ	0	105
GIN,RUM,VODKA,WHISKY 90-PROOF	1.5 F OZ	0	110
GOLDEN GRAHAMS CEREAL	1 OZ	1	110
GRAHAM CRACKER, PLAIN	2 CRACKR	1	60
GRAPE-NUTS CEREAL	1 OZ	0	100
GRAPE DRINK, CANNED	6 FL OZ	0	100
GRAPE JUICE, CANNED	1 CUP	0	155
GRAPE SODA	12 FL OZ	0	180
GRAPEFRT JCE,FRZN,CNCN UNSWTEN	6 FL OZ	1	300
GRAPEFRT JCE,FRZN,DLTD UNSWTEN	1 CUP	0	100
GRAPEFRUIT JUICE CANNED,SWTND	1 CUP	0	115
GRAPEFRUIT JUICE CANNED,UNSWT	1 CUP	0	95
GRAPEFRUIT JUICE, RAW	1 CUP	0	95
GRAPEFRUIT, CANNED SYRUP PACK	1 CUP	0	150
GRAPEFRUIT, RAW, PINK	1/2 FRUT	0	40
GRAPEFRUIT, RAW, WHITE	1/2 FRUT	0	40
GRAPEJCE,FRZN,CONCEN SWTND,W/C	6 FL OZ	1	385
GRAPEJCE,FRZN,DILUTD SWTND,W/C	1 CUP	0	125
GRAPES, EUROPEAN, RAW THOMPSN	10 GRAPE	0	35
GRAPES, EUROPEAN, RAW TOKAY	10 GRAPE	0	40
GRAVY AND TURKEY FROZEN	5 OZ	4	95
GREAT NORTHN BEANS DRY,CKD,DRN	1 CUP	1	210
GROUND BEEF, BROILED LEAN	3 OZ	16	230
GROUND BEEF, BROILED REGULAR	3 OZ	18	245
GUM DROPS	1 OZ	0	100
HADDOCK, BREADED, FRIED	3 OZ	9	175

Description of Food	Amount Per Serving	Fat (Grams)	Food Energy (Calories)
HALF AND HALF, CREAM	1 CUP	28	315
HALF AND HALF, CREAM	1 TBSP	2	20
HALIBUT, BROILED, BUTTER LEMJU	3 OZ	6	140
HAMBURGER, 4OZ PATTY	1 SANDWH	21	445
HAMBURGER, REGULAR	1 SANDWH	11	245
HARD CANDY	1 OZ	0	110
HERRING, PICKLED	3 OZ	13	190
HOLLANDAISE SCE W/ H2O,FRM MX	1 CUP	20	240
HONEY	1 CUP	0	1030
HONEY	1 TBSP	0	65
HONEY NUT CHEERIOS CEREAL	1 OZ	1	105
HONEYDEW MELON, RAW	1/10 MEL	0	45
ICE CREAM, VANLLA REGULR 11%	1 CUP	14	270
ICE CREAM, VANLLA REGULR 11%	1/2 GALN	115	2155
ICE CREAM, VANLLA REGULR 11%	3 FL OZ	5	100
ICE CREAM, VANLLA RICH 16% FT	1 CUP	24	350
ICE CREAM, VANLLA RICH 16% FT	1/2 GAL	190	2805
ICE CREAM, VANLLA SOFT SERVE	1 CUP	23	375
ICE MILK, VANILLA, 4% FAT	1 CUP	6	185
ICE MILK, VANILLA, 4% FAT	1/2 GAL	45	1470
ICE MILK, VANILLA SOFTSERV 3%	1 CUP	5	225
IMITATION CREAMERS LIQUID FRZ	1 TBSP	1	20
IMITATION CREAMERS POWDERED	1 TSP	1	10
IMITATION WHIPPED TOPPING,FRZN	1 CUP	19	240
IMITATION WHIPPED TOPPING,FRZN	1 TBSP	1	15
IMITATN SOUR DRESSING	1 CUP	39	415
IMITATN SOUR DRESSING	1 TBSP	2	20
IMITATN WHIPD TOPING PRESSRZD	1 CUP	16	185
IMITATN WHIPD TOPING PRESSRZD	1 TBSP	1	10
IMITATN WHIPD TOPING PWDRD,PRP	1 CUP	10	150

DESCRIPTION OF FOOD	AMOUNT PER SERVING	FAT (GRAMS)	FOOD ENERGY (CALORIES)
IMITATN WHIPD TOPING PWDRD,PRP	1 TBSP	0	10
ITALIAN BREAD	1 LOAF	4	1255
ITALIAN BREAD	1 SLICE	0	85
ITALIAN SALAD DRESSINGLOCAL OR	1 TBSP	0	5
ITALIAN SALAD DRESSING REGULAR	1 TBSP	9	80
JAMS AND PRESERVES	1 PKT	0	40
JAMS AND PRESERVES	1 TBSP	0	55
JELLIES	1 PKT	0	40
JELLIES	1 TBSP	0	50
JELLY BEANS	1 OZ	0	105
JERUSALEM-ARTICHOKE RAW	1 CUP	0	115
KALE, COOKED FROM FROZEN	1 CUP	1	40
KALE, COOKED FROM RAW	1 CUP	1	40
KIWIFRUIT, RAW	1 KIWI	0	45
KOHLRABI, COOKED DRAINED	1 CUP	0	50
LAMB, RIB, ROASTED LEAN ONLY	2 OZ	7	130
LAMB, RIB, ROASTED LEAN + FAT	3 OZ	26	315
LAMB,CHOPS,ARM,BRAISED LEAN	1.7 OZ	7	135
LAMB,CHOPS,ARM,BRAISED LEAN+FT	2.2 OZ	15	220
LAMB,CHOPS,LOIN,BROIL LEAN	2.3 OZ	6	140
LAMB,CHOPS,LOIN,BROIL LEAN+FAT	2.8 OZ	16	235
LAMB,LEG,ROASTED LEAN ONLY	2.6 OZ	6	140
LAMB,LEG,ROASTED LEAN+ FAT	3 OZ	13	205
LARD	1 CUP	205	1850
LARD	1 TBSP	13	115
LEMON-LIME SODA	12 FL OZ	0	155
LEMON JUICE, CANNED	1 CUP	1	50
LEMON JUICE, CANNED	1 TBSP	0	5
LEMON JUICE, RAW	1 CUP	0	60
LEMON JUICE,FRZN SINGLE-STRNGH	6 FL OZ	1	55
LEMON MERINGUE PIE	1 PIE	86	2140

Description of Food	Amount Per Serving	Fat (Grams)	Food Energy (Calories)
LEMON MERINGUE PIE	1 PIECE	14	355
LEMONADE,CONCENTRATE FRZ,UNDIL	6 FL OZ	0	425
LEMONADE,CONCEN,FRZEN DILUTED	6 FL OZ	0	80
LEMONS, RAW	1 LEMON	0	15
LENTILS, DRY, COOKED	1 CUP	1	215
LETTUCE, BUTTERHEAD RAW,HEAD	1 HEAD	0	20
LETTUCE, BUTTERHEAD RAW,LEAVE	1 LEAF	0	0
LETTUCE, CRISPHEAD RAW, HEAD	1 HEAD	1	70
LETTUCE, CRISPHEAD RAW,PIECES	1 CUP	0	5
LETTUCE, CRISPHEAD RAW,WEDGE	1 WEDGE	0	20
LETTUCE, LOOSELEAF	1 CUP	0	10
LIGHT, COFFEE OR TABLE CREAM	1 CUP	46	470
LIGHT, COFFEE OR TABLE CREAM	1 TBSP	3	30
LIMA BEANS, DRY COOKED,DRANED	1 CUP	1	260
LIMA BEANS,BABY FRZN,CKED,DRN	1 CUP	1	190
LIMA BEANS,THICK SEED FRZN,CKD	1 CUP	1	170
LIME JUICE, RAW	1 CUP	0	65
LIME JUICE,CANNED	1 CUP	1	50
LIMEADE,CONCENTRATE RZN,UNDIL	6 FL OZ	0	410
LIMEADE,CONCEN,FROZEN DILUTED	6 FL OZ	0	75
LUCKY CHARMS CEREAL	1 OZ	1	110
MACADAMIA NUTS OILRSTD, SALTED	1 CUP	103	960
MACADAMIA NUTS OILRSTD,SALTED	1 OZ	22	205
MACADAMIA NUTS OILRSTD,UNSALT	1 CUP	103	960
MACADAMIA NUTS OILRSTD,UNSALT	1 OZ	22	205
MACARONI AND CHEESE CANNED	1 CUP	10	230
MACARONI AND CHEESE HOME RCPE	1 CUP	22	430
MACARONI, COOKED, FIRM	1 CUP	1	190
MACARONI, COOKED TENDER, HOT	1 CUP	1	155
MACARONI, COOKED TENDER,COLD	1 CUP	0	115
MALT-O-MEAL, WITH SALT	1 CUP	0	120
MALT-O-MEAL, W/O SALT	1 CUP	0	120

DESCRIPTION OF FOOD	AMOUNT PER SERVING	FAT (GRAMS)	FOOD ENERGY (CALORIES)
MALTED MILK, CHOCOLATE POWDER	3/4 OZ	1	85
MALTED MILK,CHOCOLATE PWDRPPD	1 SERVNG	9	235
MALTED MILK,NATURAL POWDER	3/4 OZ	2	85
MALTED MILK,NATURAL PWDR PPRD	1 SERVNG	10	235
MANGOS, RAW	1 MANGO	1	135
MARGARINE, IMITATION 40% FAT	1 TBSP	5	50
MARGARINE, IMITATION 40% FAT	8 OZ	88	785
MARGARINE, REGULR,HARD80% FAT	1 PAT	4	35
MARGARINE, REGULR,HARD80% FAT	1 TBSP	11	100
MARGARINE, REGULR,HARD80% FAT	1/2 CUP	91	810
MARGARINE, REGULR,SOFT80% FAT	1 TBSP	11	100
MARGARINE, REGULR,SOFT80% FAT	8 OZ	183	1625
MARGARINE, SPREAD,HARD60% FAT	1 PAT	3	25
MARGARINE, SPREAD,HARD60% FAT	1 TBSP	9	75
MARGARINE, SPREAD,HARD60% FAT	1/2 CUP	69	610
MARGARINE, SPREAD,SOFT60% FAT	1 TBSP	9	75
MARGARINE, SPREAD,SOFT60% FAT	8 OZ	138	1225
MARSHMALLOWS	1 OZ	0	90
MAYONNAISE TYPE SALAD DRESSING	1 TBSP	5	60
MAYONNAISE, IMITATION	1 TBSP	3	35
MAYONNAISE, REGULAR	1 TBSP	11	100
MELBA TOAST, PLAIN	1 PIECE	0	20
MILK CHOCOLATE CANDY PLAIN	1 OZ	9	145
MILK CHOCOLATE CANDY W/ ALMOND	1 OZ	10	150
MILK CHOCOLATE CANDY W/ PENUTS	1 OZ	11	155
MILK CHOCOLATE CANDY W/ RICE C	1 OZ	7	140
MILK, LOFAT 1%, ADDED SOLIDS	1 CUP	2	105
MILK, LOFAT 1%, NO ADDEDSOLID	1 CUP	3	100
MILK, LOFAT 2%, ADDED SOLIDS	1 CUP	5	125
MILK, LOFAT 2%, NO ADDEDSOLID	1 CUP	5	120
MILK, SKIM, ADDED MILKSOLIDS	1 CUP	1	90
MILK, SKIM, NO ADDED MILKSOLID	1 CUP	0	85

DESCRIPTION OF FOOD	AMOUNT PER SERVING	FAT (GRAMS)	FOOD ENERGY (CALORIES)
MILK, WHOLE, 3.3% FAT	1 CUP	8	150
MINESTRONE SOUP, CANNED	1 CUP	3	80
MISO	1 CUP	13	470
MIXED GRAIN BREAD	1 LOAF	17	1165
MIXED GRAIN BREAD	1 SLICE	1	65
MIXED GRAIN BREAD TOASTED	1 SLICE	1	65
MIXED NUTS W/ PEANTS DRY,SALTD	1 OZ	15	170
MIXED NUTS W/ PEANTS DRY,UNSLT	1 OZ	15	170
MIXED NUTS W/ PEANTS OIL,SALTD	1 OZ	16	175
MIXED NUTS W/ PEANTS OIL,UNSLT	1 OZ	16	175
MOLASSES, CANE BLACKSTRAP	2 TBSP	0	85
MOZZARELLA CHEESE WHOLE MILK	1 OZ	6	80
MOZZARELLA CHESE,SKIM LOMOIST	1 OZ	5	80
MUENSTER CHEESE	1 OZ	9	105
MUSHROOM GRAVY CANNED	1 CUP	6	120
MUSHROOMS, CANNED DRND,W/SALT	1 CUP	0	35
MUSHROOMS, COOKED DRAINED	1 CUP	1	40
MUSHROOMS, RAW	1 CUP	0	20
MUSTARD GREENS, COOKED DRANED	1 CUP	0	20
MUSTARD, PREPARED YELLOW	1 TSP	0	5
NATURE VALLEY GRANOLA CEREAL	1 OZ	5	125
NECTARINES, RAW	1 NECTRN	1	65
NONFAT DRY MILK INSTANTIZED	1 CUP	0	245
NONFAT DRY MILK INSTANTIZED	1 ENVLPE	1	325
NOODLES, CHOW MEIN CANNED	1 CUP	11	220
NOODLES, EGG, COOKED	1 CUP	2	200
OATMEAL BREAD	1 LOAF	20	1145
OATMEAL BREAD	1 SLICE	1	65
OATMEAL BREAD, TOASTED	1 SLICE	1	65
OATMEAL W/ RAISINS COOKIES	4 COOKIE	10	245
OATMEAL,CKD,INSTNT FLVRD,FORTF	1 PKT	2	160
OATMEAL,CKD,INSTNT PLAIN,FORTF	1 PKT	2	105

DESCRIPTION OF FOOD	AMOUNT PER SERVING	FAT (GRAMS)	FOOD ENERGY (CALORIES)
OATMEAL,CKD,RG,QCK,INST W/OSAL	1 CUP	2	145
OATMEAL,CKD,RG,QCK INST,W/SALT	1 CUP	2	145
OCEAN PERCH, BREADED FRIED	1 FILLET	11	185
OKRA PODS, COOKED 8 PODS	0	25	
OLIVE OIL	1 CUP	216	1910
OLIVE OIL	1 TBSP	14	125
OLIVES, CANNED, GREEN	4 MEDIUM	2	15
OLIVES, CANNED, RIPE MISSION	3 SMALL	2	15
ONION POWDER	1 TSP	0	5
ONION RINGS, BREADED FRZN,PRPD	2 RINGS	5	80
ONION SOUP, DEHYDRATD PREPRED	1 PKT	0	20
ONION SOUP, DEHYDRTD UNPRPRED	1 PKT	0	20
ONIONS, RAW, CHOPPED	1 CUP	0	55
ONIONS, RAW, COOKED DRAINED	1 CUP	0	60
ONIONS, RAW, SLICED	1 CUP	0	40
ONIONS, SPRING, RAW	6 ONION	0	10
ORANGE JUICE, CANNED	1 CUP	0	105
ORANGE JUICE, CHILLED	1 CUP	1	110
ORANGE JUICE, RAW	1 CUP	0	110
ORANGE JUICE,FROZEN CONCENTRTE	6 FL OZ	0	340
ORANGE JUICE,FRZN,CNCN DILUTED	1 CUP	0	110
ORANGE SODA	12 FL OZ	0	180
ORANGE + GRAPEFRUIT JUCE,CANND	1 CUP	0	105
ORANGES, RAW	1 ORANGE	0	60
ORANGES, RAW, SECTIONS	1 CUP	0	85
OREGANO	1 TSP	0	5
OYSTERS, BREADED, FRIED	1 OYSTER	5	90
OYSTERS, RAW	1 CUP	4	160
PANCAKES, BUCKWHEAT FROM MIX	1 PANCAK	2	55
PANCAKES, PLAIN MIX	1 PANCAK	2	60
PANCAKES, PLAIN HOME RECIPE	1 PANCAK	2	60
PAPAYAS, RAW	1 CUP	0	65

Description of Food	Amount Per Serving	Fat (Grams)	Food Energy (Calories)
PAPRIKA	1 TSP	0	5
PARMESAN CHEESE, GRATED	1 CUP	30	455
PARMESAN CHEESE, GRATED	1 OZ	9	130
PARMESAN CHEESE, GRATED	1 TBSP	2	25
PARSLEY, FREEZE-DRIED	1 TBSP	0	0
PARSLEY, RAW	10 SPRIG	0	5
PARSNIPS, COOKED DRAINED	1 CUP	0	125
PASTERZD PROCES CHEESE SWISS	1 OZ	7	95
PASTERZD PROCES CHEESE AMERICN	1 OZ	9	105
PASTERZD PROCES CHESE FOOD,AMR	1 OZ	7	95
PASTERZD PROCES CHESE SPRED,AM	1 OZ	6	80
PEA BEANS, DRY, COOKED RAINED	1 CUP	1	225
PEACH PIE	1 PIE	101	2410
PEACH PIE	1 PIECE	17	405
PEACHES, CANNED, HEAVY SYRUP	1 CUP	0	190
PEACHES, CANNED HEAVY SYRUP	1 HALF	0	60
PEACHES, CANNED JUICE PACK	1 CUP	0	110
PEACHES, CANNED JUICE PACK	1 HALF	0	35
PEACHES, DRIED	1 CUP	1	380
PEACHES, DRIED,COOKED UNSWETND	1 CUP	1	200
PEACHES, FROZEN,SWETNED W/VITC	1 CUP	0	235
PEACHES, FROZEN,SWETNED W/VITC	10 OZ	0	265
PEACHES, RAW	1 PEACH	0	35
PEACHES, RAW, SLICED	1 CUP	0	75
PEANUT BUTTER	1 TBSP	8	95
PEANUT BUTTER COOKIE HOME RECP	4 COOKIE	14	245
PEANUT OIL	1 CUP	216	1910
PEANUT OIL	1 TBSP	14	125
PEANUTS, OIL ROASTED SALTED	1 CUP	71	840
PEANUTS, OIL ROASTED SALTED	1 OZ	14	165
PEANUTS, OIL ROASTED UNSALTED	1 CUP	71	840
PEANUTS, OIL ROASTED UNSALTED	1 OZ	14	165

Description of Food	Amount Per Serving	Fat (Grams)	Food Energy (Calories)
PEARS, CANNED HEAVY SYRUP	1 CUP	0	190
PEARS, CANNED HEAVY SYRUP	1 HALF	0	60
PEARS, CANNED, JUICE PACK	1 CUP	0	125
PEARS, CANNED, JUICE PACK	1 HALF	0	40
PEARS, RAW, BARTLETT	1 PEAR	1	100
PEARS, RAW, BOSC	1 PEAR	1	85
PEARS, RAW, D'ANJOU	1 PEAR	1	120
PEAS, EDIBLE POD, COOKED DRNED	1 CUP	0	65
PEAS, GREEN,CNND,DRND W/ SALT	1 CUP	1	115
PEAS, GREEN,CNND,DRND W/O SALT	1 CUP	1	115
PEAS, SPLIT, DRY, COOKED	1 CUP	1	230
PEAS,GRN, FROZEN COOKED DRANED	1 CUP	0	125
PEA, GREEN, SOUP, CANNED	1 CUP	3	165
PECAN PIE	1 PIE	189	3450
PECAN PIE	1 PIECE	32	575
PECANS, HALVES	1 CUP	73	720
PECANS, HALVES	1 OZ	19	190
PEPPER-TYPE SODA	12 FL OZ	0	160
PEPPERS, HOT CHILI, RAW GREEN	1 PEPPER	0	20
PEPPERS, HOT CHILI, RAW RED	1 PEPPER	0	20
PEPPERS, SWEET, COOKED GREEN	1 PEPPER	0	15
PEPPERS, SWEET, COOKED RED	1 PEPPER	0	15
PEPPERS, SWEET, RAW GREEN	1 PEPPER	0	20
PEPPERS, SWEET, RAW, RED	1 PEPPER	0	20
PEPPER, BLACK	1 TSP	0	5
PICKLES, CUCUMBER, DILL	1 PICKLE	0	5
PICKLES, CUCUMBER FRESH PACK	2 SLICES	0	10
PICKLES, CUCUMBER SWT GHERKIN	1 PICKLE	0	20
PIECRUST, FROM MIX	2 CRUST	93	1485
PIECRUST,FROM HOME RECIPE	1 SHELL	60	900
PINE NUTS	1 OZ	17	160
PINEAPPLE-GRAPEFRUIT JUICEDRNK	6 FL OZ	0	90

DESCRIPTION OF FOOD	AMOUNT PER SERVING	FAT (GRAMS)	FOOD ENERGY (CALORIES)
PINEAPPLE JUICE, CANNED UNSWTN	1 CUP	0	140
PINEAPPLE, CANNED, HEAVY SYRUP	1 CUP	0	200
PINEAPPLE, CANNED, HEAVY SYRUP	1 SLICE	0	45
PINEAPPLE, CANNED JUICE PACK	1 CUP	0	150
PINEAPPLE, CANNED JUICE PACK	1 SLICE	0	35
PINEAPPLE, RAW, DICED	1 CUP	1	75
PINTO BEANS,DRY,COOKED DRAINED	1 CUP	1	265
PISTACHIO NUTS	1 OZ	14	165
PITA BREAD	1 PITA	1	165
PIZZA, CHEESE	1 SLICE	9	290
PLANTAINS, COOKED	1 CUP	0	180
PLANTAINS, RAW	1 PLANTN	1	220
PLUMS, CANNED HEAVY SYRUP	1 CUP	0	230
PLUMS, CANNED HEAVY SYRUP	3 PLUMS	0	120
PLUMS, CANNED, JUICE PACK	1 CUP	0	145
PLUMS, CANNED, JUICE PACK	3 PLUMS	0	55
PLUMS, RAW, 1-1/2-IN DIAM	1 PLUM	0	15
PLUMS, RAW, 2-1/8-IN DIAM	1 PLUM	0	35
POPCORN, AIR-POPPED UNSALTED	1 CUP	0	30
POPCORN, POPPED, VEG OIL SALTD	1 CUP	3	55
POPCORN, SUGAR SYRUP COATED	1 CUP	1	135
POPSICLE	1 POPCLE	0	70
PORK CHOP, LOIN BROIL, LEAN	2.5 OZ	8	165
PORK CHOP, LOIN, BROIL LEAN+FT	3.1 OZ	19	275
PORK CHOP, LOIN,PANFRY LEAN	2.4 OZ	11	180
PORK CHOP, LOIN,PANFRY LEAN+FT	3.1 OZ	27	335
PORK FRESH HAM, ROASTD LEAN	2.5 OZ	8	160
PORK FRESH HAM, ROASTD LEAN+FT	3 OZ	18	250
PORK FRESH RIB, ROASTD LEAN	2.5 OZ	10	175
PORK FRESH RIB, ROASTD LEAN+FT	3 OZ	20	270
PORK SHOULDER, BRAISD LEAN	2.4 OZ	8	165
PORK SHOULDER, BRAISD LEAN+FAT	3 OZ	22	295

DESCRIPTION OF FOOD	AMOUNT PER SERVING	FAT (GRAMS)	FOOD ENERGY (CALORIES)
PORK, CURED, BACON REGUL,CKED	3 SLICE	9	110
PORK, CURED, BACON CANADN,CKED	2 SLICE	4	85
PORK, CURED, HAM CANNED,ROAST	3 OZ	7	140
PORK, CURED, HAM ROSTED,LEAN	2.4 OZ	4	105
PORK, CURED, HAM ROSTED,LN+FT	3 OZ	14	205
PORK, LINK, COOKED	1 LINK	4	50
PORK, LUNCHEON MEAT CANNED	2 SLICES	13	140
PORK, LUNCHEON MEAT CHOPPD HAM	2 SLICES	7	95
PORK, LUNCHEON MEAT CKD HAM,LN	2 SLICES	3	75
PORK, LUNCHEON MEAT CKD HAM,RG	2 SLICES	6	105
POTATO CHIPS	10 CHIPS	7	105
POTATO SALAD MADE W/ MAYONNAIS	1 CUP	21	360
POTATOES, AU GRATIN FROM MIX	1 CUP	10	230
POTATOES, AU GRATIN HOME RECP	1 CUP	19	325
POTATOES, BAKED FLESH ONLY	1 POTATO	0	145
POTATOES, BAKED WITH SKIN	1 POTATO	0	220
POTATOES, BOILED PEELED AFTER	1 POTATO	0	120
POTATOES, BOILED, PEELED BEFOR	1 POTATO	0	115
POTATOES, HASHED BROWN FR FRZN	1 CUP	18	340
POTATOES, MASHED FRM DEHYDRTED	1 CUP	12	235
POTATOES, MASHED,RECPE MLK+MAR	1 CUP	9	225
POTATOES, MASHED,RECPE W/ MILK	1 CUP	1	160
POTATOES, SCALLOPED FROM MIX	1 CUP	11	230
POTATOES, SCALLOPED HOME RECP	1 CUP	9	210
POTATOES,FRENCH-FRD FRZN,FRIED	10 STRIP	8	160
POTATOES,FRENCH-FRD FRZN,OVEN	10 STRIP	4	110
POUND CAKE, COMMERCIAL	1 LOAF	94	1935
POUND CAKE, COMMERCIAL	1 SLICE	5	110
POUND CAKE, FROM HOME RECIPE	1 LOAF	94	2025
POUND CAKE, FROM HOME RECIPE	1 SLICE	5	120
PRETZELS, STICK	10 PRETZ	0	10
PRETZELS, TWISTED, DUTCH	1 PRETZ	1	65

Description of Food	Amount Per Serving	Fat (Grams)	Food Energy (Calories)
PRETZELS, TWISTED, THIN	10 PRETZ	2	240
PRODUCT 19 CEREAL	1 OZ	0	110
PROVOLONE CHEESE	1 OZ	8	100
PRUNE JUICE, CANNED	1 CUP	0	180
PRUNES, DRIED	5 LARGE	0	115
PRUNES, DRIED, COOKED UNSWTNED	1 CUP	0	225
PUDDING, CHOCOLATE CANNED	5 OZ	11	205
PUDDING, CHOC, COOKED FROM MIX	1/2 CUP	4	150
PUDDING, CHOC, INSTANT FR MIX	1/2 CUP	4	155
PUDDING, RICE, FROM MIX	1/2 CUP	4	155
PUDDING, TAPIOCA, CANNED	5 OZ	5	160
PUDDING, TAPIOCA FROM MIX	1/2 CUP	4	145
PUDDING, VANILLA CANNED	5 OZ	10	220
PUDDING, VNLLA,COOKED FROM MIX	1/2 CUP	4	145
PUDDING, VNLLA,INSTANT FRM MIX	1/2 CUP	4	150
PUMPERNICKEL BREAD	1 LOAF	16	1160
PUMPERNICKEL BREAD	1 SLICE	1	80
PUMPERNICKEL BREAD TOASTED	1 SLICE	1	80
PUMPKIN AND SQUASH KERNELS	1 OZ	13	155
PUMPKIN PIE	1 PIE	102	1920
PUMPKIN PIE	1 PIECE	17	320
PUMPKIN, CANNED	1 CUP	1	85
PUMPKIN, COOKED FROM RAW	1 CUP	0	50
QUICHE LORRAINE	1 SLICE	48	600
RADISHES, RAW	4 RADISH	0	5
RAISIN BRAN, KELLOGG'S	1 OZ	1	90
RAISIN BRAN, POST	1 OZ	1	85
RAISIN BREAD	1 LOAF	18	1260
RAISIN BREAD	1 SLICE	1	65
RAISIN BREAD, TOASTED	1 SLICE	1	65
RAISINS	1 CUP	1	435
RAISINS	1 PACKET	0	40

DESCRIPTION OF FOOD	AMOUNT PER SERVING	FAT (GRAMS)	FOOD ENERGY (CALORIES)
RASPBERRIES, FROZEN SWEETENED	1 CUP	0	255
RASPBERRIES, FROZEN SWEETENED	10 OZ	0	295
RASPBERRIES, RAW	1 CUP	1	60
RED KIDNEY BEANS, DRY CANNED	1 CUP	1	230
REFRIED BEANS, CANNED	1 CUP	3	295
RELISH, SWEET	1 TBSP	0	20
RHUBARB, COOKED ADDED SUGAR	1 CUP	0	280
RICE KRISPIES CEREAL	1 OZ	0	110
RICE, BROWN, COOKED	1 CUP	1	230
RICE, WHITE, COOKED	1 CUP	0	225
RICE, WHITE, INSTANT COOKED	1 CUP	0	180
RICE, WHITE, PARBOILED COOKED	1 CUP	0	185
RICE, WHITE, PARBOILED RAW	1 CUP	1	685
RICE, WHITE, RAW	1 CUP	1	670
RICOTTA CHEESE, PART SKIM MILK	1 CUP	19	340
RICOTTA CHEESE WHOLE MILK	1 CUP	32	430
ROAST BEEF SANDWICH	1 SANDWH	13	345
ROLLS, DINNER COMMERCIAL	1 ROLL	2	85
ROLLS, DINNER HOME RECIPE	1 ROLL	3	120
ROLLS, FRANKFURTER + HAMBURGER	1 ROLL	2	115
ROLLS, HARD	1 ROLL	2	155
ROLLS, HOAGIE OR SUBMARINE	1 ROLL	8	400
ROOT BEER	12 FL OZ	0	165
RYE BREAD, LIGHT	1 LOAF	17	1190
RYE BREAD, LIGHT	1 SLICE	1	65
RYE BREAD, LIGHT TOASTED	1 SLICE	1	65
RYE WAFERS WHOLE-GRAIN	2 WAFERS	1	55
SAFFLOWER OIL	1 CUP	218	1925
SAFFLOWER OIL	1 TBSP	14	125
SALAMI, COOKED TYPE	2 SLICES	11	145
SALAMI, DRY TYPE	2 SLICES	7	85
SALMON, BAKED, RED	3 OZ	5	140

DESCRIPTION OF FOOD	AMOUNT PER SERVING	FAT (GRAMS)	FOOD ENERGY (CALORIES)
SALMON, CANNED, PINK W/ BONES	3 OZ	5	120
SALMON, SMOKED	3 OZ	8	150
SALT	1 TSP	0	0
SALTINES	4 CRACKR	1	50
SANDWICH SPREAD PORK, BEEF	1 TBSP	3	35
SANDWICH TYPE COOKIE	4 COOKIE	8	195
SARDINES, ATLNTC,CNNED,OIL,DRN	3 OZ	9	175
SAUERKRAUT, CANNED	1 CUP	0	45
SCALLOPS, BREADED FRZN,REHEAT	6 SCALOP	10	195
SEAWEED, KELP, RAW	1 OZ	0	10
SEAWEED, SPIRULINA, DRIED	1 OZ	2	80
SELF-RISING FLOUR UNSIFTED	1 CUP	1	440
SEMISWEET CHOCOLATE	1 CUP	61	860
SESAME SEEDS	1 TBSP	4	45
SHAKES, THICK, CHOCOLATE	10 OZ	8	335
SHAKES, THICK, VANILLA	10 OZ	9	315
SHEETCAKE W/O FRSTNG HOMERECIP	1 CAKE	108	2830
SHEETCAKE,W/ WHFRSTNG HOMERCIP	1 CAKE	129	4020
SHEETCAKE,W/ WHFRSTNG HOMERCIP	1 PIECE	14	445
SHEETCAKE,W/O FRSTNG HOMERECIP	1 PIECE	12	315
SHERBET, 2% FAT	1 CUP	4	270
SHERBET, 2% FAT	1/2 GAL	31	2160
SHORTBREAD COOKIE COMMERCIAL	4 COOKIE	8	155
SHORTBREAD COOKIE HOME RECIPE	2 COOKIE	8	145
SHREDDED WHEAT CEREAL	1 OZ	1	100
SHRIMP, CANNED, DRAINED	3 OZ	1	100
SHRIMP, FRENCH FRIED	3 OZ	10	200
SNACK CAKES,DEVILS FOOD CREMFL	SM CAKE	4	105
SNACK CAKES,SPONGE CREME FLLNG	SM CAKE	5	155
SNACK TYPE CRACKERS	1 CRACKR	1	15
SNAP BEAN,CNND,DRND GREEN,SALT	1 CUP	0	25
SNAP BEAN,CNND,DRND GRN,NOSALT	1 CUP	0	25

DESCRIPTION OF FOOD	AMOUNT PER SERVING	FAT (GRAMS)	FOOD ENERGY (CALORIES)
SNAP BEAN,CNND,DRND YLLW, SALT	1 CUP	0	25
SNAP BEAN,CNND,DRND YLLW,NOSAL	1 CUP	0	25
SNAP BEAN,FRZ,CKD,DRND GREEN	1 CUP	035	
SNAP BEAN,FRZ,CKD,DRND YELLOW	1 CUP	0	35
SNAP BEAN,RAW,CKD,DRND GREEN	1 CUP	0	45
SNAP BEAN,RAW,CKD,DRND YELLOW	1 CUP	0	45
SOUR CREAM	1 CUP	48	495
SOUR CREAM	1 TBSP	3	25
SOY SAUCE	1 TBSP	0	10
SOYBEAN-COTTONSEED OIL HYDRGN	1 CUP	218	1925
SOYBEAN-COTTONSEED OIL HYDRGN	1 TBSP	14	125
SOYBEAN OIL HYDROGENATED	1 CUP	218	1925
SOYBEAN OIL HYDROGENATED	1 TBSP	14	125
SOYBEANS, DRY, COOKED DRAINED	1 CUP	10	235
SPAGHETTI, COOKED, FIRM	1 CUP	1	190
SPAGHETTI, COOKED TENDER	1 CUP	1	155
SPAGHETTI, TOM SAUCE CHEES,CND	1 CUP	2	190
SPAGHETTI, TOM SAUCE CHEE,HMRP	1 CUP	9	260
SPAGHETTI,MEATBALLS TOMSAC,CND	1 CUP	10	260
SPAGHETTI,MEATBALLS TOMSA,HMRP	1 CUP	12	330
SPECIAL K CEREAL	1 OZ	0	110
SPINACH SOUFFLE	1 CUP	18	220
SPINACH, CANNED DRND,W/ SALT	1 CUP	1	50
SPINACH, CANNED, DRND W/O SALT	1 CUP	1	50
SPINACH, COOKED FR FRZEN, DRND	1 CUP	0	55
SPINACH, COOKED FROM RAW, DRND	1 CUP	0	40
SPINACH, RAW	1 CUP	0	10
SQUASH, SUMMER COOKED, DRAIND	1 CUP	1	35
SQUASH, WINTER, BAKED	1 CUP	1	80
STRAWBERRIES, FROZEN SWEETEND	1 CUP	0	245
STRAWBERRIES, FROZEN SWEETEND	10 OZ	0	275
STRAWBERRIES, RAW	1 CUP	1	45

DESCRIPTION OF FOOD	AMOUNT PER SERVING	FAT (GRAMS)	FOOD ENERGY (CALORIES)
SUGAR COOKIE, FROM REFRIG DOGH	4 COOKIE	12	235
SUGAR FROSTED FLAKES KELLOGG	1 OZ	0	110
SUGAR SMACKS CEREAL	1 OZ	1	105
SUGAR, BROWN, PRESSED DOWN	1 CUP	0	820
SUGAR, POWDERED, SIFTED	1 CUP	0	385
SUGAR, WHITE GRANULATED	1 CUP	0	770
SUGAR, WHITE GRANULATED	1 PKT	0	25
SUGAR, WHITE GRANULATED	1 TBSP	0	45
SUNFLOWER OIL	1 CUP	218	1925
SUNFLOWER OIL	1 TBSP	14	125
SUNFLOWER SEEDS	1 OZ	14	160
SUPER SUGAR CRISP CEREAL	1 OZ	0	105
SWEET (DARK) CHOCOLATE	1 OZ	10	150
SWEETENED CONDENSED MILK CNND	1 CUP	27	980
SWEETPOTATOES, BAKED PEELED	1 POTATO	0	115
SWEETPOTATOES, BOILED W/O PEEL	1 POTATO	0	160
SWEETPOTATOES, CANDIED	1 PIECE	3	145
SWEETPOTATOES, CANNED MASHED	1 CUP	1	260
SWEETPOTATOES, CNNED VAC PACK	1 PIECE	0	35
SWISS CHEESE	1 OZ	8	105
SYRUP, CHOCOLATE FLAVORED THIN	2 TBSP	0	85
SYRUP, CHOCOLATE FLVRED, FUDGE	2 TBSP	5	125
TABLE SYRUP (CORN AND MAPLE)	2 TBSP	0	122
TACO	1 TACO	11	195
TAHINI	1 TBSP	8	90
TANGERINE JUICE CANNED,SWTNED	1 CUP	0	125
TANGERINES, CANNED LIGHT SYRP	1 CUP	0	155
TANGERINES, RAW	1 TANGRN	0	35
TARTAR SAUCE	1 TBSP	8	75
TEA, BREWED	8 FL OZ	0	0
TEA, INSTANT,PREPRD UNSWEETEND	8 FL OZ	0	0
TEA,INSTANT,PREPARD SWEETENED	8 FL OZ	0	85

DESCRIPTION OF FOOD	AMOUNT PER SERVING	FAT (GRAMS)	FOOD ENERGY (CALORIES)
TOASTER PASTRIES	1 PASTRY	6	210
TOFU	1 PIECE	5	85
TOMATO JUICE, CANNED WITH SALT	1 CUP	0	40
TOMATO JUICE CANNED W/O SALT	1 CUP	0	40
TOMATO PASTE, CANNED WITH SALT	1 CUP	2	220
TOMATO PASTE, CANNED W/O SALT	1 CUP	2	220
TOMATO PUREE CANNED WITH SALT	1 CUP	0	105
TOMATO PUREE, CANNED W/O SALT	1 CUP	0	105
TOMATO SAUCE, CANNED WITH SALT	1 CUP	0	75
TOMATO SOUP WITH MILK CANNED	1 CUP	6	160
TOMATO SOUP W/ WATER CANNED	1 CUP	2	85
TOMATO VEG SOUP DEHYD,PREPRED	1 PKT	1	40
TOMATOES, CANNED S+L, W/ SALT	1 CUP	1	50
TOMATOES, CANNED S+L,W/O SALT	1 CUP	1	50
TOMATOES, RAW	1 TOMATO	0	25
TORTILLAS, CORN	1 TORTLA	1	65
TOTAL CEREAL	1 OZ	1	100
TRIX CEREAL	1 OZ	0	110
TROUT, BROILED W/ BUTTR,LEMJU	3 OZ	9	175
TUNA SALAD	1 CUP	19	375
TUNA, CANND, DRND,OIL CHK,LGHT	3 OZ	7	165
TUNA, CANND, DRND WATR, WHITE	3 OZ	1	135
TURKEY HAM, CURED TURKEY THIGH	2 SLICES	3	75
TURKEY LOAF, BREAST MEAT W/O C	2 SLICES	1	45
TURKEY LOAF, BREAST MEAT, W/ C	2 SLICES	1	45
TURKEY PATTIES, BRD BATTD,FRID	1 PATTY	12	180
TURKEY ROAST, FRZN LGHT+DRK,CK	3 OZ	5	130
TURKEY, ROASTED, DARK MEAT	4 PIECES	6	160
TURKEY, ROASTED LIGHT MEAT	2 PIECES	3	135
TURKEY, ROASTED LIGHT + DARK	1 CUP	7	240
TURKEY, ROASTED LIGHT + DARK	3 PIECES	4	145
TURNIP GREENS, CKED FRM FROZEN	1 CUP	1	50

301

DESCRIPTION OF FOOD	AMOUNT PER SERVING	FAT (GRAMS)	FOOD ENERGY (CALORIES)
TURNIP GREENS, COOKED FROM RAW	1 CUP	0	30
TURNIPS, COOKED, DICED	1 CUP	0	30
VANILLA WAFERS	10 COOKE	7	185
VEAL CUTLET, MED FAT BRSD,BRLD	3 OZ	9	185
VEAL RIB, MED FAT ROASTED	3 OZ	14	230
VEGETABLE BEEF SOUP CANNED	1 CUP	2	80
VEGETABLE JUICE COCKTAIL, CNND	1 CUP	0	45
VEGETABLES, MIXED CANNED	1 CUP	0	75
VEGETABLES, MIXED CKED FR FRZ	1 CUP	0	105
VEGETARIAN SOUP CANNED	1 CUP	2	70
VIENNA BREAD	1 SLICE	1	70
VIENNA SAUSAGE	1 SAUSAG	4	45
VINEGAR AND OILSALAD DRESSING	1 TBSP	8	70
VINEGAR, CIDER	1 TBSP	0	0
WAFFLES, FROM HOME RECIPE	1 WAFFLE	13	245
WAFFLES, FROM MIX	1 WAFFLE	8	205
WALNUTS, BLACK, CHOPPED	1 CUP	71	760
WALNUTS, BLACK, CHOPPED	1 OZ	16	170
WALNUTS, ENGLISH, PIECES	1 CUP	74	770
WALNUTS, ENGLISH, PIECES	1 OZ	18	180
WATER CHESTNUTS, CANNED	1 CUP	0	70
WATERMELON, RAW	1 PIECE	2	155
WATERMELON, RAW, DICED	1 CUP	1	50
WHEAT BREAD	1 LOAF	19	1160
WHEAT BREAD	1 SLICE	1	65
WHEAT BREAD, TOASTED	1 SLICE	1	65
WHEAT FLOUR ALL-PURPOSE,SIFTD	1 CUP	1	420
WHEAT FLOUR ALL-PURPOSE,UNSIF	1 CUP	1	455
WHEATIES CEREAL	1 OZ	0	100
WHEAT, THIN CRACKERS	4 CRACKR	1	35
WHIPPED TOPPING PRESSURIZED	1 CUP	13	155
WHIPPED TOPPING PRESSURIZED	1 TBSP	1	10

Description of Food	Amount Per Serving	Fat (Grams)	Food Energy (Calories)
WHIPPING CREAM UNWHIPED,HEAVY	1 CUP	88	820
WHIPPING CREAM UNWHIPED,HEAVY	1 TBSP	6	50
WHIPPING CREAM UNWHIPED,LIGHT	1 CUP	74	700
WHIPPING CREAM UNWHIPED,LIGHT	1 TBSP	5	45
WHITE BREAD	1 LOAF	18	1210
WHITE BREAD CRUMBS,SOFT	1 CUP	2	120
WHITE BREAD CUBES	1 CUP	1	80
WHITE BREAD, SLICE 18 PER LOAF	1 SLICE	1	65
WHITE BREAD, SLICE 22 PER LOAF	1 SLICE	1	55
WHITE BREAD, TOASTED 18 PER	1 SLICE	1	65
WHITE BREAD, TOASTED 22 PER	1 SLICE	1	55
WHITE CAKE W/ WHT FRSTNG,COMML	1 CAKE	148	4170
WHITE CAKE W/WHT FRSTNG,COMML	1 PIECE	9	260
WHITE SAUCE W/ MILK FROM MIX	1 CUP	13	240
WHITE SAUCE, MEDIUM HOME RECP	1 CUP	30	395
WHOLE-WHEAT BREAD	1 LOAF	20	1110
WHOLE-WHEAT BREAD	1 SLICE	1	70
WHOLE-WHEAT BREAD TOASTED	1 SLICE	1	70
WHOLE-WHEAT FLOUR HRD WHT,STIR	1 CUP	2	400
WHOLE-WHEAT WAFERS CRACKERS	2 CRACKR	2	35
WINE, DESSERT	3.5 F OZ	0	140
WINE, TABLE, RED	3.5 F OZ	0	75
WINE, TABLE, WHITE	3.5 F OZ	0	80
YEAST, BAKERS, DRY ACTIVE	1 PKG	0	20
YEAST, BREWERS, DRY	1 TBSP	0	25
YELLOW CAKE W/ CHOC FRST,FRMIX	1 CAKE	125	3735
YELLOW CAKE W/ CHOC FRST,FRMIX	1 PIECE	8	235
YELLOWCAKE W/ CHOCFRSTNG,COMML	1 CAKE	175	3895
YELLOWCAKE W/ CHOCFRSTNG,COMML	1 PIECE	11	245
YOGURT, W/ LOFAT MILK, PLAIN	8 OZ	4	145
YOGURT, W/ LOFAT MILK FRUITFLV	8 OZ	2	230

Description of Food	Amount Per Serving	Fat (Grams)	Food Energy (Calories)
YOGURT, W/ NONFAT MILK	8 OZ	0	125
YOGURT, W/ WHOLE MILK	8 OZ	7	140

(The preceding food data is provided by "Nutritional Chart Copyright Health Advantage/Mike Vincitorio http://www.ntwrks.com/~mikev Raw data provided by the U.S. Department of Agriculture.")

FAST-FOOD REFERENCE GUIDE

Since such a large part of the American diet is from eating outside the home, I have included this "Fast Food" listing of some of the major fast-food restaurants. This can be especially helpful when trying to quickly evaluate and determine just what and where to eat while at your desk or in your car.

Again, only the total calorie and fat gram content of each food will be given, which is still at this time, our only concern.

Arby's

	Calories	Fat Grams
BACON	90	7
BISCUIT (PLAIN)	280	15
BLUEBERRY MUFFIN	230	9
CINNAMON NUT DANISH	360	11
CROISSANT (PLAIN)	220	12
EGG PORTION	95	8
FRENCH TOASTIX (6)	430	21
HAM	45	1
SAUSAGE	163	15
SWISS CHEESE	45	3
TABLE SYRUP	100	0
ARBY'S MELT W/CHEDDAR	368	18
ARBY-Q	431	18
BAC'N CHEDDAR DELUXE	539	34
BEEF'N CHEDDAR	487	28
GIANT ROAST BEEF	555	28
JUNIOR ROAST BEEF	324	14
REG. ROAST BEEF	388	19
SUPER ROAST BEEF	523	27
BREADED CHICKEN FILLET	536	28
CHICKEN CORDON BLEU	623	33
CHICKEN FINGERS (2)	290	16
GRILLED CHICKEN BBQ	388	13
GRILLED CHICKEN DELUXE	430	20
ROAST CHICKEN CLUB	546	31
ROAST CHICKEN DELUXE	433	22
ROAST CHICKEN SANTA FE	436	22
FRENCH DIP	475	22

	Calories	Fat Grams
HOT HAM'N SWISS	500	23
ITALIAN SUB	675	36
PHILLY BEEF'N SWISS	755	47
ROAST BEEF SUB	700	42
TRIPLE CHEESE MELT	720	45
TURKEY SUB	550	27
ROAST BEEF DELUXE	296	10
ROAST CHICKEN DELUXE	276	6
ROAST TURKEY DELUXE	260	7
GARDEN SALAD	61	0.5
ROAST CHICKEN SALAD	149	2
SIDE SALAD	23	0.3
FISH FILLET	529	27
HAM 'N CHEESE	359	14
HAM 'N CHEESE MELT	329	13
CHEDDAR CURLY FRIES	333	18
CURLY FRIES	300	15
FRENCH FRIES	246	13
POTATO CAKES	204	12
BAKED POTATO (PLAIN)	355	0.3
BAKED POTATO W/SOUR CREAM/MARG	578	24
BROCCOLI 'N CHEDDAR BAKED POTATO	571	20
DELUXE BAKED POTATO	736	36
BOSTON CLAM CHOWDER (WHOLE MILK)	190	9
CREAM OF BROCCOLI (WHOLE MILK)	160	8
LUMBERJACK MIXED VEGETABLE	90	4
OLD FASHIONED CHICKEN NOODLE	80	2
POTATO WITH BACON (WHOLE MILK)	170	7
TIMBERLINE CHILI	220	10
WISCONSIN CHEESE (WHOLE MILK)	280	18
APPLE TURNOVER	330	14
CHERRY TURNOVER	320	13
CHEESECAKE (PLAIN)	320	23
CHOCOLATE CHIP COOKIE	125	6
CHOCOLATE SHAKE	451	12
JAMOCHA SHAKE	384	10
VANILLA SHAKE	360	12
BUTTERFINGER POLAR SWIRL	457	18
HEATH POLAR SWIRL	543	22
OREO POLAR SWIRL	482	22
PEANUT BUTTER CUP POLAR SWIRL	517	24
SNICKERS POLAR SWIRL	511	19
2% MILK	5	0
COCA-COLA CLASSIC	140	0
COFFEE	3	0
DIET COKE	0	0

	Calories	Fat Grams
DIET PEPSI	0	0
DIET SEVEN UP	0	0
DR. PEPPER	160	0
HOT CHOCOLATE	110	1
ICED TEA	6	0
NEHI ORANGE	195	0
ORANGE JUICE	82	0
PEPSI COLA	150	0
RC COLA	165	0
RC DIET RITE	1	0
SEVEN UP	144	0
UPPER TEN	169	0
ARBY'S SAUCE	15	0.2
BEEF STOCK AU JUS	10	0
BARBECUE SAUCE	30	0
BLEU CHEESE DRESSING	290	31
CHEDDAR CHEESE SAUCE	35	3
HONEY FRENCH DRESSING	280	23
HORSEY SAUCE	60	5
KETCHUP	16	0
LT. CHOLESTEROL FREE MAYONNAISE	12	1
MAYONNAISE	110	12
MUSTARD, GERMAN STYLE	5	0
NON-SEPARATING ITALIAN SUB SAUCE	70	7
PARMESAN CHEESE SAUCE	70	7
RED RANCH DRESSING	75	6
REDUCED CALORIE HONEY MAYO	70	7
REDUCED CALORIE ITALIAN DRESSING	20	1
REDUCED CALORIE BUTTERMILK RANCH	50	0
TARTAR SAUCE	140	15
THOUSAND ISLAND DRESSING	260	26

BOSTON MARKET

	Calories	Fat Grams
1/4 WHITE MEAT CHICKEN NO SKIN/WING	160	3.5
1/4 WHITE MEAT CHICKEN W/SKIN	330	17
1/4 DARK MEAT CHICKEN NO SKIN	210	10
1/4 DARK MEAT CHICKEN W/SKIN	330	22
1/2 CHICKEN WITH SKIN	630	37
SKINLESS ROTISSERIE TURKEY BREAST	170	1
HAM W/CINNAMON APPLES	350	13
MEATLOAF/CHUNKY TOMATO SAUCE	370	18
MEATLOAF/BROWN GRAVY	390	22
ORIG. CHICKEN POT PIE	750	34
CHUNKY CHICKEN SALAD	390	30
CAESER SALAD ENTRÉE	520	43

	Calories	Fat Grams
CAESER SALAD NO DRESSING	240	13
CHICKEN CAESER SALAD	670	47
CHICKEN SOUP	80	3
CHICKEN TORTILLA SOUP	220	11
CHICKEN SANDWICH W/CHEESE & SAUCE	760	32
CHICKEN SANDWICH (PLAIN)	430	3.5
CHICKEN SALAD SANDWICH	680	33
TURKEY SANDWICH W/CHEESE & SAUCE	710	28
TURKEY SANDWICH (PLAIN)	400	3.5
HAM SANDWICH W/CHEESE & SAUCE	760	35
HAM SANDWICH (PLAIN)	450	9
MEATLOAF SANDWICH W/CHEESE	860	33
MEATLOAF (PLAIN)	690	21
HAM/TURKEY CLUB W/CHEESE & SAUCE	890	43
HAM/TURKEY CLUB (PLAIN)	430	6
STEAMED VEGETABLES	35	0.5
NEW POTATOES	140	3
BUTTERED CORN	190	4
ZUCCHINI MARINARA	80	4
MASHED POTATOES	180	8
HOMESTYLE MASHED POTATOES & GRAVY	200	9
CHICKEN GRAVY	15	1
RICE PILAF	180	5
CREAMED SPINACH	300	24
STUFFING	310	12
BUTTERNUT SQUASH	160	6
MACARONI & CHEESE	280	10
BBQ BAKED BEANS	330	9
HOT CINNAMON APPLES	250	4.5
FRUIT SALAD	70	0.5
MED. PASTA SALAD	170	10
CRANBERRY RELISH	370	5
COLE SLAW	280	16
TORTELLINI SALAD	380	24
CAESER SIDE SALAD	210	17
CORN BREAD	200	6
OATMEAL RAISIN COOKIE	320	13
CHOCOLATE CHIP COOKIE	340	17
BROWNIE	450	27

BASKIN ROBBINS

	Calories	Fat Grams
NON FAT CHOCOLATE VANILLA TWIST	100	0
DAIQUIRI ICE	110	0
RED RASBERRY SORBET	120	0
TROPIC OF FRUIT NON FAT YOGURT	130	0

	Calories	Fat Grams
ESPRESSO 'N CREAM	110	4
RAINBOW SHERBET	120	1.5
MAUI BROWNIE MADNESS	140	3
PERILS OF PRALINE	130	3
RASBERRY CHEESE LOUISE	130	3
CHOCOLATE CHOCOLATE CHIP (NO SUGAR)	100	2.5
THIN MINT (NO SUGAR)	100	2.5
SILK CHOCOLATE	120	0
VANILLA BEAN DREAM	120	0
DUTCH CHOCOLATE	100	0
STRAWBERRY NON FAT YOGURT	100	0
VANILLA BEAN DREAM NON FAT YOGURT	110	0
CAFÉ MOCHA YOGURT	80	0
CHOCOLATE YOGURT	80	0
VANILLA YOGURT	80	0
CHOCOLATE ICE CREAM	150	8
CHOCOLATE CHIP ICE CREAM	150	9
ROCKY ROAD ICE CREAM	160	8
VANILLA ICE CREAM	140	8
VERY BERRY STRAWBERRY ICE CREAM	120	6
TROPICAL TANGO SMOOTHIE	180	0
BORA BERRY BORA SMOOTHIE	170	0
COPA BANANA SMOOTHIE	140	0
ALOHA BERRY BANANA SMOOTHIE	160	0
CALYPSO BERRY SMOOTHIE	160	0
SUNSET ORANGE SMOOTHIE	150	0

BRUEGGER'S

	Calories	Fat Grams
TURKEY LENTIL SUPERB	140	1.8
TERRIFIC TURKEY ORZO	93	2.7
THE BIG CHILL	203	5.6
CAJUN GUMBO	104	2
VICTORY GARDEN VEGGIE	76	1.6
MARCELLO MINESTRONE	75	1.8
VELVET VEGGIE CHEESE	205	11.3
CHILE CILANTRO	195	6.1
GARDEN SPLIT PEA	194	4.6
RATATOUILLE	142	9.1
CLAM CHOWDER	164	5.7
AZTEC CHICKEN	97	2.4
CHICKEN NOODLE	112	2.6
BACON & CORN CHOWDER	192	8.3
PLAIN	280	1.5
HONEY GRAIN	290	2
CINNAMON RAISIN	290	1.5

	Calories	Fat Grams
PUMPERNICKEL	280	1.5
POPPY	280	1.5
SESAME	290	2.5
SALT	280	1.5
ONION	280	1.5
GARLIC	280	1.5

BURGER KING

	Calories	Fat Grams
WHOPPER SANDWICH	640	39
WHOPPER SANDWICH WITH CHEESE	730	46
DOUBLE WHOPPER	870	56
DOUBLE WHOPPER WITH CHEESE	960	63
WHOPPER JR	420	24
WHPPER JR WITH CHEESE	460	28
HAMBURGER	330	15
CHEESEBURGER	380	19
DOUBLE CHEESEBURGER	600	36
DOUBLE CHEESEBURGER WITH BACON	640	39
BK BIG FISH	700	41
BK BROILER	550	29
CHICKEN SANDWICH	710	43
CHICKEN TENDERS (8 PIECE)	310	17
BROILED CHICKEN SALAD	200	10
GARDEN SALAD NO DRESSING	100	5
SIDE SALAD NO DRESSING	60	3
FRENCH FRIES (MED./SALTED)	370	20
COATED FRENCH FRIES (MED./SALTED)	340	17
ONION RINGS	310	14
DUTCH APPLE PIE	300	15
VANILLA SHAKE (MED)	300	6
CHOCOLATE SHAKE (MED)	320	7
CHOCOLATE SHAKE (MED/SYRUP ADDED)	440	7
STRAWBERRY SHAKE (MED/SYRUP ADDED)	420	6
COCA COLA CLASSIC (MED)	280	0
DIET COKE (MED)	1	0
SPRITE (MED)	260	0
TROPICANA ORANGE JUICE	140	0
COFFEE	5	0
MILK - 2% LOW FAT	130	5
CROISSAN'WICH W/SAUSAGE, EGG, CHEESE	600	46
BISCUIT W/SAUSAGE	590	40
BISCUIT W/BACON, EGG, CHEESE	510	31
FRENCH TOAST STICKS	500	27
HASH BROWNS	220	12
A.M. EXPRESS GRAPE JAM	30	0

	Calories	Fat Grams
A.M. EXPRESS STRAWBERRY JAM	30	0
PROC. AM. CHEESE	90	8
LETTUCE	0	0
TOMATO	5	0
ONION	5	0
PICKLES	0	0
KETCHUP	15	0
MUSTARD	0	0
MAYONNAISE	210	23
TARTAR SAUCE	180	19
LAND O' LAKES WHIPPED CLASSIC BLEND	65	7
BULL'S EYE BBQ SAUCE	20	0
BACON BITS	15	1
CROUTONS	30	1
1000 ISLAND	140	12
FRENCH	140	10
RANCH	180	19
BLEU CHEESE	160	16
RED. CAL LT. ITALIAN	15	0.5
A.M. EXPRESS DIP	80	0
HONEY	90	0
RANCH	170	17
BBQ	35	0
SWEET/SOUR	45	0

DAIRY QUEEN

	Calories	Fat Grams
DQ VANILLA SOFT SERVE, 1/2 CUP	140	4.5
DQ CHOCOLATE SOFT SERVE, 1/2 CUP	150	5
DQ NONFAT FROZEN YOGURT, 1/2 CUP	100	0
SMALL VANILLA CONE	230	7
REGULAR VANILLA CONE	350	10
LARGE VANILLA CONE	410	12
SMALL CHOCOLATE CONE	240	8
REGULAR CHOCOLATE CONE	360	11
REGULAR YOGURT CONE	280	1
SMALL CHOCOLATE SUNDAE	290	7
REGULAR CHOCOLATE SUNDAE	410	10
REGULAR CUP OF YOGURT	230	0.5
REGULAR YOGURT STRAWBERRY SUNDAE	300	0.5
SMALL MISTY SLUSH	0	0
REGULAR MISTY SLUSH	290	0
STRAWBERRY MISTY COOLER	190	0
SMALL CHOCOLATE MALT	650	16
REGULAR CHOCOLATE MALT	880	22
SMALL CHOCOLATE SHAKE	560	15

	Calories	Fat Grams
REGULAR CHOCOLATE SHAKE	770	20
DQ SANDWICH	150	5
STRAWBERRY SHORTCAKE	430	14
BANANA SPLIT	510	12
CHOCOLATE DILLY BAR	210	13
CHOCOLATE MINT DILLY BAR	190	12
TOFFEE DILLY BAR WITH HEATH PIECES	210	12
FUDGE NUT BAR	410	25
BUSTER BAR	450	28
PEANUT BUSTER PARFAIT	730	31
SMALL DIPPED CONE	340	17
REGULAR DIPPED CONE	510	25
STARKISS	80	0
DQ CARAMEL & NUT BAR	260	13
DQ FUDGE BAR	50	0
DQ VANILLA ORANGE BAR	60	0
DQ LEMON FREEZ'R, 1/2 CUP	80	0
SMALL BUTTERFINGER BLIZZARD	520	18
REGULAR BUTTERFINGER BLIZZARD	750	26
SM. CHOC. SAND. COOKIE BLIZZARD	520	18
REG. CHOC. SAND. COOKIE BLIZZARD	640	23
SMALL STRAWBERRY BLIZZARD	400	11
REGULAR STRAWBERRY BLIZZARD	570	16
SMALL HEATH BLIZZARD	560	21
REGULAR HEATH BLIZZARD	820	33
SM. CHOC. CHIP COOKIE DOUGH BLIZZARD	660	24
REG. CHOC. CHIP COOKIE DOUGH BLIZZARD	950	36
SM. REESE'S PEANUT BUTTER CUP BLIZZARD	590	24
REG. REESE'S PEANUT BUTTER CUP BLIZZARD	790	33
SM. STRAWBERRY BREEZE	320	0.5
REG. STRAWBERRY BREEZE	460	1
SMALL HEATH BREEZE	470	10
REGULAR HEATH BREEZE	710	18
QUEEN'S CHOICE VANILLA BIG SCOOP	250	14
QUEEN'S CHOICE CHOCOLATE BIG SCOOP	250	14
STRAWBERRY-BANANA DQ TREATZZA PIZZA (1/8)	180	6
HEATH DQ TREATZZA PIZZA (1/8)	180	7
M&M DQ TREATZZA PIZZA (1/8)	190	7
PEANUT BUTTER FUDGE DQ TREATZZA PIZZA (1/8)	220	10
DQ FROZEN LOG CAKE (1/8)	280	9
DQ FROZEN 8" ROUND CAKE (1/8)	340	12
DQ FROZEN 10" ROUND CAKE (1/12)	360	12
DQ FROZEN HEART CAKE (1/10)	270	9
DQ FROZEN SHEET CAKE (1/20)	350	12

DOMINO'S

	Calories	Fat Grams
HAND TOSSED CHEESE (2/12)	319	10
THIN CRUST CHEESE (1/6)	255	11
DEEP DISH CHEESE (2/12)	464	20
HAND TOSSED GR PEPPERS,OLIVES,MUSHROOM (2/12)	335	11
THIN CRUST GR PEPPERS,OLIVES,MUSHROOMS (1/6)	271	12
DEEP DISH GR PEPPERS,OLIVES,MUSHROOMS (2/12)	479	21
HAND TOSSED PEPPERONI,ITALIAN SAUSAGE (2/12)	418	18
THIN CRUST PEPPERONI,ITALIAN SAUSAGE (1/6)	354	19
DEEP DISH PEPPERONI,ITALIAN SAUSAGE (2/12)	563	28
HAND TOSSED CHEESE (2/8)	350	10.5
THIN CRUST CHEESE (1/4)	273	11.5
DEEP DISH CHEESE (2/8)	466	21.5
HAND TOSSED GR PEPPERS,OLIVES,MUSHROOMS (2/8)	368	12
THIN CRUST GR PEPPERS,OLIVES,MUSHROOMS (1/4)	292	13
DEEP DISH GR PEPPERS,OLIVES,MUSHROOMS (2/8)	486	28
HAND TOSSED PEPPERONI,ITALIAN SAUSAGE (2/8)	466	20.5
THIN CRUST PEPPERONI,ITALIAN SAUSAGE (1/4)	390	21.5
DEEP DISH PEPPERONI,ITALIAN SAUSAGE (2/8)	583	31
CHEESE PIZZA (1 PIZZA)	591	27
GR PEPPERS,OLIVES,MUSHROOMS (1 PIZZA)	605	28
PEPPERONI,ITALIAN SAUSAGE (1 PIZZA)	685	35
BARBEQUE WINGS	50	25
HOT WINGS	45	2.5
BREADSTICKS (1)	77	3
CHEESY BREAD (1)	103	5.5
SMALL GARDEN SALAD	22	0.3
LARGE GARDEN SALAD	39	0.5
THOUSAND ISLAND	200	20
HONEY FRENCH	210	18
LT. ITALIAN	20	1
HOUSE ITALIAN	220	24
BLEU CHEESE	220	24
RANCH	260	29
FF RANCH	40	0
CREAMY CAESER	200	22

GODFATHER'S PIZZA

	Calories	Fat Grams
ORIGINAL CRUST MINI 1/4	131	3
ORIGINAL CRUST MEDIUM 1/8	231	5
ORIGINAL CRUST LARGE 1/10	258	6
ORIGINAL CRUST JUMBO 1/10	382	9
ORIGINAL CRUST MINI 1/4	176	7
ORIGINAL CRUST MEDIUM 1/8	306	11

	Calories	Fat Grams
ORIGINAL CRUST LARGE 1/10	338	12
ORIGINAL CRUST JUMBO 1/10	503	18
GOLDEN CRUST MEDIUM 1/8	212	8
GOLDEN CRUST LARGE 1/10	242	9
GOLDEN CRUST MEDIUM 1/8	271	12
GOLDEN CRUST LARGE 1/10	305	14

HARDEE'S

	Calories	Fat Grams
RISE 'N' SHINE BISCUIT	390	21
JELLY BISCUIT	440	21
APPLE CINNAMON 'N' RAISIN BISCUIT	200	8
SAUSAGE BISCUIT	510	31
SAUSAGE/EGG BISCUIT	630	40
BACON/EGG BISCUIT	570	33
BACON/EGG/CHEESE BISCUIT	610	37
HAM BISCUIT	400	20
HAM/EGG/CHEESE BISCUIT	540	30
COUNTRY HAM BISCUIT	430	22
BIG COUNTRY SAUSAGE	1000	66
BIG COUNTRY BACON	820	49
FRISCO HAM SANDWICH	500	25
REG HASH ROUNDS (16)	230	14
BISCUIT 'N' GRAVY	510	28
THREE PANCAKES	280	2
ULTIMATE OMELET BISCUIT	570	33
ORANGE JUICE (12 OZ)	140	0
HAMBURGER	270	11
CHEESEBURGER	310	14
THE BOSS	570	33
CRAVIN' BACON CHEESEBURGER	690	46
THE WORKS BURGER	530	30
MESQUITE BACON CHEESEBURGER	370	18
QUARTER POUND DBL. CHEESEBURGER	470	27
CHICKEN FILLET SANDWICH	480	18
REG ROAST BEEF	320	16
BIG ROAST BEEF	460	24
GRILLED CHICKEN	350	11
MUSHROOM 'N' SWISS BURGER	490	25
FRISCO SANDWICH	720	46
HOT HAM 'N' CHEESE	310	12
FISHERMAN'S FILLET	560	27
BREAST	370	15
WING	200	8
THIGH	330	15
LEG	170	7

	Calories	Fat Grams
COLE SLAW (4 OZ)	240	20
MASHED POTATOES (4 OZ)	70	N/A
GRAVY (1.5 OZ)	20	N/A
BAKED BEANS (SM. - 5 OZ)	170	1
SIDE SALAD	25	N/A
GARDEN SALAD	220	13
GRILLED CHICKEN SALAD	150	3
FF FRENCH DRESSING	70	0
RANCH DRESSING	290	29
THOUSAND ISLAND DRESSING	250	23
FRENCH FRIES (SMALL)	240	10
FRENCH FRIES (MEDIUM)	350	15
FRENCH FRIES (LARGE)	430	18
VANILLA SHAKE	350	5
CHOCOLATE SHAKE	370	5
STRAWBERRY SHAKE	420	4
PEACH SHAKE	390	4
VANILLA CONE	170	2
CHOCOLATE CONE	180	2
COOL TWIST CONE	180	2
HOT FUDGE SUNDAE	290	6
STRAWBERRY SUNDAE	210	2
PEACH COBBLER (SM - 6 OZ)	310	7
BIG COOKIE	280	12

KFC

	Calories	Fat Grams
WING WITH SKIN	121	8
BREAST WITH SKIN	251	11
BREAST WITHOUT SKIN	169	4
THIGH WITH SKIN	207	12
THIGH WITHOUT SKIN	106	5.5
DRUMSTICK WITH SKIN	97	4
DRUMSTICK WITHOUT SKIN	67	2.5
WHOLE WING	140	10
BREAST	400	24
DRUMSTICK	140	9
THIGH	250	18
WHOLE WING	200	13
BREAST	470	28
DRUMSTICK	190	11
THIGH	370	25
WHOLE WING	210	15
BREAST	530	35
DRUMSTICK	190	11
THIGH	370	27

	Calories	Fat Grams
3 CRISPY STRIPS	261	16
CHUNKY CHICKEN POT PIE	770	42
HOT WINGS PIECES (6)	471	33
ORIGINAL RECIPE CHICKEN SANDWICH	497	22
VALUE BBQ CHICKEN SANDWICH	256	8
KENTUCKY NUGGETS (6)	284	18
CORN ON THE COB	190	3
GREEN BEENS	45	1.5
BBQ BAKED BEANS	190	3

LEEANN CHIN

	Calories	Fat Grams
CREAM CHEESE PUFFS	331	29
SHRIMP TOAST	150	11
EGGROLLS	210	11
CHINESE CHICKEN SALAD LARGE	191	10
CHINESE SALAD DRESSING	135	9
LEMON CHICKEN W/SAUCE	260	12
LEEANN LITE CHICKEN & VEGETABLES	128	5
SICHUAN NOODLES W/VEGETABLES	276	18
PEKING CHICKEN	510	35
VEGETABLE FRIED RICE	181	7
SPICY CHICKEN W/ZUCCHINI	214	9
SHRIMP W/VEGETABLES	428	9

MCDONALD'S

	Calories	Fat Grams
HAMBURGER	260	9
CHEESEBURGER	320	13
QUARTER POUNDER	420	21
QUARTER POUNDER W/CHEESE	530	30
BIG MAC	560	31
ARCH DELUXE	550	31
ARCH DELUXE W/BACON	590	34
CRISPY CHICKEN DELUXE	500	25
FISH FILLET DELUXE	560	28
GRILLED CHICKEN DELUXE	440	20
SMALL	210	10
LARGE	450	22
SUPER	540	26
CHICKEN MCNUGGETS 4	190	11
CHICKEN MCNUGGETS 6	290	17
CHICKEN MCNUGGETS 9	430	26
HOT MUSTARD	60	3.5
BARBECUE SAUCE	45	0
SWEET 'N SOUR SAUCE	50	0

	Calories	Fat Grams
HONEY	45	0
HONEY MUSTARD	50	4.5
LIGHT MAYONNAISE	40	4
GARDEN SALAD	35	0
GRILLED CHICKEN SALAD DELUXE	120	1.5
CROUTONS	50	1.5
CAESAR	160	14
FF HERB VIN	50	0
RANCH	230	21
RED FRENCH RED CAL	160	8
EGG MCMUFFIN	290	12
SAUSAGE MCMUFFIN	360	23
SAUSAGE MCMUFFIN W/EGG	440	28
ENGLISH MUFFIN	140	2
SAUSAGE BISCUIT	430	29
SAUSAGE BISCUIT/EGG	510	35
BACON/EGG/CHEESE BISCUIT	440	26
BISCUIT	260	13
SAUSAGE	170	16
SCRAMBLED EGGS (2)	160	11
HASH BROWNS	130	8
HOTCAKES PLAIN	310	7
HOTCAKES W/MARGARINE & SYRUP	580	16
BREAKFAST BURRITO	320	20
LOWFAT APPLE BRAN MUFFIN	300	3
APPLE DANISH	360	16
CHEESE DANISH	410	22
CINNAMON ROLL	400	20
VANILLA RED FAT CONE	150	4.5
STRAWBERRY SUNDAE	290	7
HOT CARAMEL SUNDAE	360	10
HOT FUDGE SUNDAE	340	12
NUTS SUNDAE	40	3.5
BAKED APPLE PIE	260	13
CHOCOLATE CHIP COOKIE	170	10
MCDONALDLAND COOKIES	180	5
VANILLA SHAKE SMALL	360	9
CHOCOLATE SHAKE SMALL	360	9
STRAWBERRY SHAKE SMALL	360	9
1% LOWFAT MILK	100	2.5
ORANGE JUICE	80	0
COCA-COLA CHILD	110	0
COCA-COLA SMALL	150	0
COCA-COLA MEDIUM	210	0
COCA-COLA LARGE	310	0
DIET COKE CHILD	0	0

	Calories	Fat Grams
DIET COKE SMALL	0	0
DIET COKE MEDIUM	0	0
DIET COKE LARGE	0	0
SPRITE CHILD	110	0
SPRITE SMALL	150	0
SPRITE MEDIUM	210	0
SPRITE LARGE	310	0
HI-C ORANGE CHILD	120	0
HI-C ORANGE SMALL	160	0
HI-C ORANGE MEDIUM	240	0
HI-C ORANGE LARGE	350	0

PIZZA HUT

	Calories	Fat Grams
THIN 'N CRISPY	210	9
HAND TOSSED	280	10
PAN	300	14
STUFFED CRUST	380	11
THIN 'N CRISPY	240	11
HAND TOSSED	280	10
PAN	310	14
STUFFED CRUST	410	14
THIN 'N CRISPY	190	6
HAND TOSSED	230	6
PAN	250	9
STUFFED CRUST	380	14
THIN 'N CRISPY	220	9
HAND TOSSED	260	9
PAN	280	12
STUFFED CRUST	410	17
THIN 'N CRISPY	300	16
HAND TOSSED	300	12
PAN	350	18
STUFFED CRUST	430	19
THIN 'N CRISPY	270	13
HAND TOSSED	290	11
PAN	300	13
STUFFED CRUST	420	16
THIN 'N CRISPY	310	16
HAND TOSSED	290	11
PAN	360	19
STUFFED CRUST	500	23
THIN 'N CRISPY	170	6
HAND TOSSED	240	7
PAN	240	9
STUFFED CRUST	390	14

	Calories	Fat Grams
THIN 'N CRISPY	270	12
HAND TOSSED	320	13
PAN	350	17
STUFFED CRUST	480	22
THIN 'N CRISPY	250	11
HAND TOSSED	270	9
PAN	300	13
STUFFED CRUST	440	16
THIN 'N CRISPY	280	13
HAND TOSSED	290	10
PAN	340	16
STUFFED CRUST	470	20
THIN 'N CRISPY	220	7
HAND TOSSED	240	6
PAN	280	11
STUFFED CRUST	390	13
PEPPERONI	670	29
SUPREME	710	31
CHEESE	630	24
BUFFALO WINGS MILD (5)	200	12
BUFFALO WINGS HOT (4)	210	12
GARLIC BREAD (1 SLICE)	150	8
BREAD STICK (1 SLICE)	130	4
BREAD STICK DIP SAUCE	30	0.5
SPAGHETTI W/MARINARA	490	6
SPAGHETTI W/MEAT SAUCE	600	13
SPAGHETTI W/MEATBALLS	850	24
CAVATINI PASTA	480	14
CAVATINI SUPREME PASTA	560	19
HAM & CHEESE SANDWICH	550	21
SUPREME SANDWICH	640	28
APPLE DESSERT PIZZA (1 SLICE)	250	4.5
CHERRY DESSERT PIZZA (1 SLICE)	250	4.5

RAX

	Calories	Fat Grams
REG RAX	388	22
DELUXE	521	35
BBC	716	51
GRILLED CHICKEN	526	33
JR. DELUXE	367	25
BBQ BEEF	399	19.5
MUSHROOM MELT	599	37.5
TURK/BACON CLUB	680	46.5
TURKEY	484	32
CHEDDAR MELT	346	23

	Calories	Fat Grams
PHILLY MELT	537	32
PLAIN	207	0
CHEESE/BROCCOLI	281	0.2
CHEESE	270	0.2
CHEESE/BACON	336	18.5
BUTTER	306	11
SOUR TOPPING	257	4
CREAM OF BROCCOLI	95	4
CHICKEN NOODLE	113	1
CHILI	158	9.5
VANILLA	220	0.5
CHOCOLATE	210	0.5
STRAWBERRY	300	0.5
GRILLED CHICKEN CAESER	160	5
CAESER SIDE	40	2
SIDE	40	4
GOURMET	220	9
FF RANCH	32	0
FF ITALIAN	12	0
FF CATALINA	32	0
BUTTERMILK RANCH	175	20
BLUE CHEESE	145	16
1000 ISLAND	130	13
HONEY FRENCH	140	5
VINAIGRETTE	30	2
CREAMY CAESER	140	15
REG RAX	305	13
DELUXE	326	13
GRILLED CHICKEN	283	7
JR. DELUXE	215	8
BBQ BEEF	316	10
TURKEY	233	4
CHEDDAR MELT	283	15.5
PLAIN	207	0
CHEESE/BROCCOLI	281	0.2
CHEESE	270	0.2
BUTTER	306	11
SOUR TOPPING	257	4
CREAM OF BROCCOLI	95	4
CHICKEN NOODLE	113	1
CHILI	158	9.5
VANILLA YOGURT	220	0.5
CHOCOLATE YOGURT	310	0.5
STRAWBERRY YOGURT	300	0.5
GRILLED CHICKEN CAESER	160	5
CAESER SIDE	40	2

	Calories	Fat Grams
SIDE	40	4
GOURMET	220	9
FF RANCH	32	0
FF ITALIAN	12	0
FF CATALINA	32	0
HONEY FRENCH	140	5
VINAIGRETTE	30	2
CREAMY CAESER	140	15

SUBWAY

	Calories	Fat Grams
VEGGIE DELITE WHITE	222	3
VEGGIE DELITE WHEAT	237	3
TURKEY WHITE	273	4
TURKEY WHEAT	289	4
COLD CUT TRIO WHITE	362	13
COLD CUT TRIO WHEAT	378	13
HAM WHITE	287	5
HAM WHEAT	302	5
SUBWAY CLUB WHITE	297	5
SUBWAY CLUB WHEAT	312	5
STEAK & CHEESE WHITE	383	10
STEAK & CHEESE WHEAT	398	10
ROAST BEEF WHITE	288	5
ROAST BEEF WHEAT	303	5
SPICY ITALIAN WHITE	467	24
SPICY ITALIAN WHEAT	482	25
TURKEY BREAST & HAM WHITE	280	5
TURKEY BREAST & HAM WHEAT	295	5
CLASSIC ITALIAN B.M.T. WHITE	445	21
CLASSIC ITALIAN B.M.T. WHEAT	460	22
TUNA WHITE	527	32
TUNA WHEAT	542	32
SUBWAY SEAFOOD & CRAB WHITE	415	19
SUBWAY SEAFOOD & CRAB WHEAT	430	19
ROASTED CHICKEN BREAST WHITE	332	6
ROASTED CHICKEN BREAST WHEAT	348	6
SUBWAY MELT WHITE	366	12
SUBWAY MELT WHEAT	382	12
MEATBALL WHITE	404	16
MEATBALL WHEAT	419	16
CHICKEN TACO SUB WHITE	421	16
CHICKEN TACO SUBWAY WHEAT	436	16
PIZZA SUB WHITE	448	22
PIZZA SUB WHEAT	464	22
B.L.T. WHITE	311	10

	Calories	Fat Grams
B.L.T. WHEAT	327	10
CHOCOLATE CHIP (1 COOKIE)	210	10
OATMEAL RAISIN (1 COOKIE)	200	8
PEANUT BUTTER (1 COOKIE)	220	12
CHOCOLATE CHIP/M&M (1 COOKIE)	210	10
CHOCOLATE CHUNK (1 COOKIE)	210	10
SUGAR (1 COOKIE)	230	12
WHITE CHIP MACADEMIA NUT (1 COOKIE)	230	12
BRAZIL NUT & CHOCOLATE CHIPS (1 COOKIE)	230	12
ONIONS	5	0
LETTUCE	4	0
TOMATOES (2 SLICES)	6	0
PICKLES (3 CHIPS)	2	0
PEPPERS (2 STRIPS)	1	0
OLIVES (2 RINGS)	2	0
BACON (2 SLICES)	45	4
CHEESE (2 TRIANGLES)	41	3
LIGHT MAYONNAISE (1 TSP.)	18	2
MAYONNAISE (1 TSP.)	37	4
OIL (1 TSP.)	45	5
MUSTARD (2 TSP.)	8	0
VINEGAR (1 TSP.)	1	0
TURKEY	235	4
HAM	234	4
ROAST BEEF	245	4
BOLOGNA	292	12
SUBWAY SEAFOOD & CRAB	298	11
TUNA	354	18
VEGGIE DELITE	51	1
TURKEY BREAST	102	2
SUBWAY CLUB	126	3
SUBWAY SEAFOOD & CRAB	244	17
TUNA (LIGHT)	205	13
ROASTED CHICKEN BREAST	162	4
COLD CUT TRIO	191	11

TACO BELL

	Calories	Fat Grams
TACO	170	10
SOFT TACO	210	10
TACO SUPREME	220	13
SOFT TACO SUPREME	260	14
DOUBLE DECKER TACO	340	15
DOUBLE DECKER SUPREME	390	18
STEAK SOFT TACO	200	7
BLT SOFT TACO	340	23

	Calories	Fat Grams
KID'S SOFT TACO ROLL-UP	290	16
BEAN	380	12
BURRITO SUPREME	440	18
BIG BEEF SUPREME	520	23
7-LAYER	540	24
CHILI CHEESE	330	13
CHICKEN CLUB	540	31
BACON CHEESEBURGER	560	30
TOSTADA	300	14
MEXICAN PIZZA	570	36
BIG BEEF MEXIMELT	300	16
TACO SALAD W/SALSA	840	52
TACO SALAD W/SALSA NO SHELL	420	21
CHEESE QUESADILLA	370	20
CHICKEN QUESADILLA	420	22
STEAK FAJITA	460	21
CHICKEN FAJITA	460	21
VEGGIE FAJITA	420	19
STEAK FAJITA SUPREME	510	25
CHICKEN FAJITA SUPREME	500	25
VEGGIE FAJITA SUPREME	460	23
LT. CHICKEN	310	8
LT. CHICKEN SUPREME	430	13
LT. CHICKEN SOFT TACO	180	5
LT. KID'S CHICKEN SOFT TACO	180	5
NACHOS	310	18
BIG BEEF NACHOS SUPREME	430	24
NACHOS BELLGRANDE	740	39
PINTOS 'N CHEESE	190	8
MEXICAN RICE	190	10
CINNAMON TWISTS	140	6
GREEN SAUCE	5	0
GUACAMOLE	35	3
HOT TACO SAUCE	0	0
MILD TACO SAUCE	0	0
NACHO CHEESE SAUCE	120	10
PICANTE SAUCE	0	0
PICO DE GALLO	5	0
RED SAUCE	10	0
SALSA	25	0
CHEDDAR CHEESE	30	2
PEPPER JACK CHEESE	25	2
SOUR CREAM	40	4
NON-FAT SOUR CREAM	20	0
FF CHEDDAR CHEESE	10	0
PEPSI-COLA	200	0

	Calories	Fat Grams
DIET PEPSI	0	0
MOUNTAIN DEW	227	0
SLICE	200	0
DR. PEPPER	208	0
LIPTON BRISK ICED TEA UNSWEETENED	0	0
LIPTON BRISK ICED TEA SWEETENED	140	0
COFFEE	5	0
2% LOWFAT MILK	110	4.5
ORANGE JUICE	80	0
FIESTA BURRITO	280	16
COUNTRY BURRITO	270	14
GRANDE BURRITO	420	22
DBL. BACON/EGG BURRITO	480	27
BREAKFAST CHEESE QUESADILLA	390	22
BREAKFAST QUESADILLA W/BACON	460	28
BREAKFAST QUESADILLA W/SAUSAGE	440	26

TACO JOHN'S

	Calories	Fat Grams
BEAN BURRITO	329	N/A
BEEF BURRITO	335	N/A
CHICKEN FAJITA BURRITO	298	N/A
CHICKEN FAJITA SOFT-SHELL	200	N/A
TACO BRAVO	333	N/A
TACO BURGER	283	N/A
CRISPY TACO	184	N/A
SOFT-SHELL TACO	232	N/A
SIERRA CHICKEN FILLET SANDWICH	N/A	N/A
COMBO BURRITO	N/A	N/A
RANCH BURRITO	N/A	N/A
SUPER BURRITO	N/A	N/A
KID'S MEAL, CRISPY TACO	N/A	N/A
KID'S MEAL, SOFT-SHELL TACO	N/A	N/A
MEXI ROLLS W/SOUR CREAM	N/A	N/A
MEXI ROLLS W/GUACAMOLE	N/A	N/A
"REFRIED" BEANS	301	N/A
TEXAS CHILI	297	N/A
CHICKEN FAJITA SALAD	216	N/A
NACHOS W/CHEESE	294	N/A
NACHO CHEESE	80	N/A
HOUSE SALAD DRESSING	114	N/A
SALSA	21	N/A
SOUR CREAM	30	N/A
MEXICAN STYLE RICE	N/A	N/A
POTATO OLE'S, REGULAR	N/A	N/A
POTATO OLE'S, LARGE	N/A	N/A

	Calories	Fat Grams
POTATO OLE'S, BRAVO	N/A	N/A
POTATO OLE'S W/NACHO CHEESE	N/A	N/A
TACO SALAD	256	N/A
CHOCO TACO	320	N/A
CHURRO	147	N/A
FLAUTA, APPLE	85	N/A
FLAUTA, CHERRY	143	N/A
FLAUTA, CREAM CHEESE	181	N/A

WENDY'S

	Calories	Fat Grams
CHICKEN CAESER PITA	490	18
CLASSIC GREEK PITA	440	20
GARDEN RANCH CHICKEN PITA	480	18
GARDEN VEGGIE PITA	400	17
PLAIN SINGLE	350	15
SINGLE W/EVERYTHING	440	23
BIG BACON CLASSIC	640	36
JR. HAMBURGER	270	9
JR. CHEESEBURGER	320	13
JR. BACON CHEESEBURGER	440	25
JR. CHEESEBURGER DELUXE	390	20
HAMBURGER KIDS' MEAL	270	9
CHEESEBURGER KIDS' MEAL	310	13
GRILLED CHICKEN SANDWICH	290	7
BREADED CHICKEN SANDWICH	450	20
CHICKEN CLUB SANDWICH	520	25
1/4 LB HAMBURGER	190	12
JR. HAMBURGER	90	6
GRILLED CHICKEN FILLET	100	2.5
BREADED CHICKEN FILLET	220	10
KAISER BUN	190	3
SANDWICH BUN	160	2.5
AMERICAN CHEESE	70	6
AMERICAN CHEESE JR.	45	4
BACON	30	2.5
KETCHUP	10	0
LETTUCE	0	0
MAYONNAISE	70	7
MUSTARD	0	0
ONION	0	0
PICKLES	0	0
RED. CAL. HONEY MUSTARD	25	1.5
TOMATOES	5	0
APPLESAUCE	30	0
BACON BITS	40	1.5

	Calories	Fat Grams
BROCCOLI	0	0
CANTALOUPE, SLICED	15	0
CARROTS	5	0
CAULIFLOWER	0	0
CHEDDAR CHIPS	70	4
CHEESE, SHREDDED	50	4
CHICKEN SALAD	70	5
CHIVES	0	0
CHOW MEIN NOODLES	35	2
COLE SLAW	45	3
COTTAGE CHEESE	30	1.5
CROUTONS	30	1
CUCUMBERS	0	0
EGGS, HARD COOKED	40	3
GREEN PEAS	15	0
GREEN PEPPERS	0	0
HONEYDEW, SLICED	20	0
JALAPENO PEPPERS	0	0
ICEBERG LETTUCE	10	0
MUSHROOMS	0	0
OLIVES, BLACK	15	1.5
ORANGE, SECTIONED	10	0
PASTA SALAD	25	0
PEACHES, SLICED	15	0
PEPPERONI, SLICED	30	3
PINEAPPLE, CHUNKED	20	0
POTATO SALAD	80	7
PUDDING, CHOC	70	3
PUDDING, VANILLA	70	3
RED ONIONS	0	0
SEAFOOD SALAD	70	4
SESAME BREADSTICK	15	0
STRAWBERRIES	10	0
STRAWBERRY BANANA DESSERT	30	0
SUNFLOWER SEEDS/RAISINS	80	5
TOMATO WEDGED	5	0
TURKEY HAM DICED	50	4
WATERMELON WEDGED	20	0
SMALL	240	12
MEDIUM	340	17
BIGGIE	420	20
PLAIN	310	0
BACON & CHEESE	530	18
BROCCOLI & CHEESE	460	14
CHEESE	560	23
CHILI & CHEESE	610	24

	Calories	Fat Grams
SOUR CREAM & CHIVES	380	6
SOUR CREAM	60	6
WHIPPED MARGARINE	60	5
SMALL	190	6
LARGE	290	9
CHEDDAR CHEESE	70	6
SALTINE CRACKERS	25	0.5
6 PIECE	280	20
BBQ SAUCE	50	0
HONEY	45	0
SWEET/SOUR SAUCE	45	0
SWEET MUSTARD SAUCE	50	1
CHOC CHIP COOKIE	270	11
FROSTY DAIRY SMALL	340	10
FROSTY DAIRY MEDIUM	460	13
FROSTY DAIRY LARGE	570	17
COLA, SMALL	90	0
DIET COLA SMALL	0	0
LEMON-LIME SMALL	90	0
LEMONADE, SMALL	90	0
COFFEE	0	0
DECAF COFFEE	0	0
HOT CHOCOLATE	9	1
TEA, HOT	0	0
TEA, ICED	0	0
MILK, 2%	110	4

WHITE CASTLE

	Calories	Fat Grams
HAMBURGER	135	7
CHEESEBURGER	160	9
DBL. HAMBURGER	235	14
DBL. CHEESEBURGER	285	18
BACON CHEESEBURGER	200	13
FISH SANDWICH	160	6
CHICKEN SANDWICH	190	8
BREAKFAST SANDWICH	340	25
CHICKEN RINGS	310	21
ONION CHIPS	180	9
FRENCH FRIES	115	6
CHEESE STICKS	290	17
COCA-COLA	120	N/A
DIET COKE	1	N/A
COFFEE	6	N/A
ICED TEA	45	N/A
CHOCOLATE SHAKE	220	7

(The preceding figures have been extracted from the Internet at consumer.ag@state.mn.us., based on the book "Fast Food Facts" by the consumer division of the Minnesota Attorney Generals' office.)

Updated information can usually be found free via the Internet, related books, or simply by asking the restaurant directly.